Women/Cancer/Fear/Power series, volume 1

CANCER AS A WOMEN'S ISSUE

Women/Cancer/Fear/Power series, volume 1

CANCER AS A WOMEN'S ISSUE

Scratching the Surface

Midge Stocker, editor

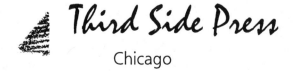 *Third Side Press*

Chicago

Cover art by E.G. Crichton.
  First published in *Out/Look Magazine*, spring 1988.
Cover design by Loraine Edwalds
Text design and production by Midge Stocker

We gratefully acknowledge the following for permission to reprint previously published work:

JACKIE WINNOW: "Lesbians Evolving Health Care" appeared in *Sinister Wisdom 39: On Disability* (winter 1989–1990) and in edited form in *Out/Look*, No. 5 (summer 1989) as "Lesbians Working on AIDS: Assessing the Impact on Health Care for Women." Reprinted by permission of the author.

NICKY MORRIS: "Legacy" appeared in *Sojourner*. Reprinted by permission of the author.

RITA ARDITTI: "CAUTION: IVF May Be Harmful to Your Health" appeared in *Reproductive and Genetic Engineering: Journal of International Feminist Analysis,* vol. 3, no. 3, 1990 (Pergamon Press). Reprinted by permission of the author.

SELMA MIRIAM: A portion of "Thoughts on Cancer and Healing" appeared in *The Second Seasonal Political Palate* (Bridgeport, CT: Sanguinaria Publishers, 1984). Reprinted by permission of the author.

ISBN: 1-879427-01-X Women/Cancer/Fear/Power series
ISBN: 1-879427-02-8 volume 1 (Cancer as a Women's Issue)

Library of Congress Cataloging-in-Publication Data

Cancer as a women's issue : scratching the surface / Midge Stocker, editor.
     p. cm. - - (Women/cancer/fear/power series ; v. 1)
     Includes bibliographical references and index
     ISBN 1-879427-02-8 : $10.95
     1. Cancer - - Social aspects. 2. Women - - Diseases. 3. Cancer - - Psychological aspects. 4. Cancer - - Political aspects.   I. Stocker, Midge, 1960 - . II. Series.
RC281.W65C35 1991
362.1'9994'0082 - - dc20   91-8809
                                                      CIP

This book is available on tape to disabled women from the Womyn's Braille Press, P.O. Box 8475, Minneapolis, MN 55408.

Third Side Press
2250 W. Farragut
Chicago, IL 60625-1802

First edition, May 1991
10 9 8 7 6 5 4 3 2 1

362.19
C215

To the survivors,
living and dead.

May we be mindful
of your example.

Contents

Introduction *by Midge Stocker*   *1*

Ripening: A Path to Cancer Activism
    by Helen Ramirez Odell   9

Lesbians Evolving Health Care: Our
    Lives Depend on It *by Jackie Winnow*   23

No Big Deal *by Jane Murtaugh*   37

Thoughts on Cancer & Healing
    by Selma Miriam   47

From a Cancer Journal *by Merida Wexler*   53

Fighting Spirit *by Nancy Lanoue*   59

My Body: A Map of Memories *by Ada
    Harrigan*   69

Changes: The Before and the After
    by Beverly Lickteig Loder   77

CAUTION: IVF May Be Harmful
    to Your Health *by Rita Arditti*   85

Lifestyles Don't Kill. Carcinogens in
    Air, Food, and Water Do.: Imagining
    Political Responses to Cancer
    by Sandra Steingraber   91

One Day At a Time: Excerpts from
    a Journal *by Rita Arditti*   103

Air Born *by Portia Cornell*   129

Live and Let Live *by Laura Post* 135

Legacy *by Nicky Morris* 143

Real Life? *by Wendy Ann Ryden* 147

Hostile Takeovers *by Naomi Glauberman* 159

White Flowers and a Grizzly Bear:
  Finding New Metaphors
  by Dian Marino 183

Fear of Cancer *by Carol Gloor* 197

Afterword *by Midge Stocker* 198

Resources 199

Contributors 202

Index 207

Introduction

Midge Stocker

Many people ask me why I decided to publish this book. There are several answers. It is personal: I want to avenge my losses. It is political: I want to fight for a better future.

In this anthology you hear the voices of real women, heterosexual and lesbian, whose lives have been changed by the experience of cancer in themselves or another. They speak to you in the hope that they can help make your journey a little easier or more meaningful, to let you know that you are not alone. If you have cancer yourself, if you fear that you have cancer and are afraid to go to the doctor and find out, if you are struggling with the fear and pain of the cancer of a loved one, you are not alone.

The Personal

We all have our stories; that is part of the problem. Nearly every woman knows, has known, or will know someone with cancer. When those people die, the tragedy is often compounded by its effect on those left behind. We hear all too often of the young mother who dies leaving young children behind. Nicky Morris is the daughter ("Legacy," pages 143–146) of a mother whose fear of dying of cancer was so great that she put Nicky and her sister into an orphanage. Wendy Ann Ryden writes of her experience of caring for her own mother during the dying process ("Real Life?" pages 147–158). Nancy Lanoue describes the character of survivorship in "Fighting Spirit" (pages 59–68) as she talks about her experience with breast cancer followed by her partner's experience with pancreatic cancer. My own stories are perhaps less dramatic; nonetheless they impel me to look for more stories and for change that can reduce the number of sad stories to be told.

1

As coordinator of the Writers Conference at the National Women's Music Festival, one of my jobs is to invite featured speakers and make arrangements for their accommodations. Over the past few years, three of the well-known women writers who had agreed to appear at the festival were unable to attend because of health reasons—all three have had cancer: Pat Parker, Audre Lorde, and May Sarton. And Pat Parker died in June 1989 at the age of 45—a major loss for the world of poetry and life. As I had these encounters with Pat Parker, Audre Lorde, and May Sarton, I began to feel increasingly anxious about inviting featured speakers: whose illness would I find out about next?

2

I am a survivor of childhood sexual abuse. The incident of this abuse that I remember most clearly involves a man who was my French horn teacher for a few months. His decision to molest me changed my life, strongly influencing my decision to drop my plans to become a professional musician (although I had been accepted as a student by several major con-servatories). After he molested me, I became unable to enjoy music. Eventually, I tried to reintegrate music into my life.

In the fall of 1983, I met a woman who played the piano; Rue had played the trombone but was unable to continue doing that because of the stoma left after her laryngectomy for throat cancer. We became friends and decided to try playing together once a week.

I began to regather my ability to play horn, and my memories. Rue was dealing with her loss too; she would much rather have been playing brass duets with me. The winter was hard for her, and in the spring she went into the hospital for what she thought would be a few days. I left town on business for a week. I returned home to a message on my answering machine from her partner. My friend had died while I was away, and they were hoping I would get back in time to play horn at the funeral. I was too late. I stopped playing again.

3

In the summer of 1986, my mother's older brother married a young woman named Lynn. Lynn was a remarkable woman, the sort of woman with whom everyone immediately feels comfortable. She was the sort of person who makes everyone feel included in a group and everyone welcome in her home. She was the sort of person who could bring together people who had previously seemed distant from one another and make us feel like family. She overcame resistance from family members and made us love her.

Within a week after the wedding, Lynn was diagnosed with breast cancer. She had felt for the preceding six months that something was wrong and had consulted several doctors, all of whom assured her nothing was. The mammogram taken six months before had been read to show no problem (upon later examination, the cancer was clearly present in the film). Within a month after the wedding, Lynn had a radical mastectomy. She followed a course of chemotherapy through the fall, followed by radiation in the winter. The doctors were very encouraging. They had done their job, they thought, and were holding out the hope for her that she could soon bear a child. Lynn was preparing for reconstructive surgery in the spring when the doctors determined that they had been wrong. The cancer had metastasized to her liver.

Lynn was in an experimental program and tried every treatment available to her. She was as well cared for as a woman could be. Her father, mother, sister, and brothers are all doctors; they watched out for her. She had bone marrow removed before radiation treatment for later implantation. She followed an intensive treatment program. She survived through the summer and into the early fall, managing even to go on a scuba diving trip in September. And she died at the beginning of October. She was 35.

When it seemed clear that her time was limited by cancer, I made the decision not to get to know her better. I did not want to reduce in any way the time or strength she would have to spend with those who knew her better and who would feel her loss even more deeply than I.

Yet I feel her absence often. And I am angry.

4

Loraine, who was my partner for many years, is the middle of seven children. Her mother worked full time as a nurse while raising those children. When the youngest of the children were finally in college, her mother was diagnosed with inoperable lung cancer. That was more than ten years ago now, and that woman's children have barely begun to recover from the loss.

5

When I finally began to be able to talk about cancer, one of the first people I talked with was Jane Murtaugh (whose story "No Big Deal" appears on pages 37–46). Jane is a survivor of four different kinds of cancer over a period of seven years that ended in August 1985. I want to know why that happened to her. Why she got sick, and why she got well. And why many other women do not.

The Political

The work of collecting manuscripts for this book comes from my anger and my desire to learn more about the problem. It has taken me a long time to be able to grieve the losses I have experienced. I have been spurred along by articles that appeared in *Sojourner* in the fall of 1989 and by reports that some kind of women's cancer support group was being formed in Boston. "What a great idea!" I thought, having the idea reinforced by reading Sonny Wainwright's description of the Lesbian Illness-Support Group that helped her through the process of cancer treatment in New York City in the early 1980s.[*]

Why do women need books, groups, support programs of our own? It's true, of course, that men get cancer. (I'm especially aware of this because my grandfather was diagnosed with prostate cancer while I was collecting manuscripts for this book.) It's also true that treatments for cancer are tested primarily on men—and presumably work better, or at least more predictably, on them. And, according to the American Cancer Society's estimates for 1990, gender-linked cancers are far more common among

---

[*] Sonny Wainwright, *Stage V: A Journal Through Illness* (Berkeley, CA: Acacia Books, 1984).

women (combined estimate for new cases of breast,
uterine, and ovarian cancers: 251,500; deaths from
these cancers, 67,300) than among men (estimated
new cases of prostate cancer: 106,000; deaths,
30,000). Moreover, the incidence of breast cancer,
particularly among young women, is on the rise,
with the statistics having been adjusted in 1987 to
one in ten and then to one in nine in 1991. What will
that rate be by 1995?

Cancer affects women differently than it does
men. One reason is that our support systems are constructed differently. When a man gets sick, it is
nearly always a woman who takes care of him—usually a wife, sometimes a mother or daughter,
occasionally a hired caregiver. This is true even of
gay men. With the onset of the AIDS epidemic, support systems for gay men sprang up out of nowhere;
they are relatively well funded, due to the fact that
the primary affected population was initially white,
male, and affluent. Many of the workers in those
support systems are women; many, as Jackie Winnow discusses in her article "Lesbians Evolving
Health Care" (pages 23–36) are lesbians, working on
behalf of what used to be called "gay liberation" and
what is now called the "lesbian and gay movement":
our name gets added to the title and our energy
sapped away from our own work.

Women need to pay attention to our own needs.
When we get sick, who takes care of us? Most of the
time it is our mothers, sisters, daughters, women
with whom we have significant relationships. If we
live independently, as single women or as single
mothers, our layer of possible supporters may be
particularly thin. Women in the lesbian community
have vastly fewer resources than heterosexual
women do. Lesbians are always classified as single
women. Accordingly, lesbians (and other single

women) as a group have a fairly low standard of living, as a result of the sexist employment paradigm in the United States. If men make nearly twice as much money (even for doing the same work) as women do, on average, then (assuming that both are in coupled relationships) a heterosexual woman is likely to be a member of a household that has more money available to it than does a lesbian in whose household there is no male income—one male income plus one female income is greater than two female incomes (by far!). From this perspective, gay men do well—two male incomes equal at least three, and probably close to four, times two female incomes—which helps explain why so many resources have been activated in support of people with AIDS. Moreover, lesbians and gay men, no matter how committed their relationships, share the dilemma of not being able to benefit from employee benefits—like health insurance—of their spouses as heterosexual couples who are married can. Lesbians start out poor and when we get sick we get poorer.

For women who choose alternative lifestyles of any kind, for women who want to explore alternatives to the prescriptions and proscriptions of Western medicine, for women who do not fit the mold prescribed by the likes of *Cosmopolitan*, *Redbook*, and *Ladies' Home Journal*, the mainstream groups that have been established for women with cancer may cause as much pain as they alleviate. As Nancy Lanoue suggests ("Fighting Spirit," pages 59–68), the mainstream idea of a normal range of motion may differ significantly from ours. As Sandra Steingraber points out ("Lifestyles Don't Kill. Carcinogens in Air, Food, and Water Do.: Imagining Political Responses to Cancer," pages 91–102), we need groups that affirm our right to make our own choices, of all kinds. Grassroots organizations working around women and cancer are now springing up around the country—in Boston, Oakland, Washington, Chicago, and Los Angeles. Perhaps you can start a group in your area. Do what you can. Start by talking.

Ripening: A Path to Cancer Activism

Helen Ramirez Odell

About ten years ago, I met Meridel Le Sueur at a reception in honor of the publication of her writings in a new edition of *Ripening*.* We talked about the women's movement and unions; she expressed her wish that garment workers all over the world would earn decent wages due to global organizing. I was struck by the fact that she was so alert and focused on the future even though she was over 80 years old. I thought most people her age spent their days talking and thinking about the past. That night I vowed that I too would still be planning and working for a better future when I was 80 years old. At 40 I was in excellent health and felt invincible. Little did I know that I may not make it to my eighties.

As a nurse and a feminist, I was interested in women's health issues. I delighted in the progress women made in regaining control over the birth process and the surroundings in which birth took place. I deplored the injuries women suffered due to the Dalkon Shield and was pleased that women took action by filing legal claims against A.H. Robbins. When my doctor recommended a mammogram as part of my routine checkup I refused.

At that time, the American Cancer Society and the National Cancer Institute disagreed as to whether women my age should have them. The whole subject of the diagnosis and treatment of breast cancer

---

* Meridel Le Sueur, *Ripening: Selected Work, 1927–1980,* New York: The Feminist Press, 1982.

was a controversial one, and I was leery of the benefits of mammography compared to the risks. Although mammography had been improved so that the radiation dosage was low, I was aware that the cumulative effect of x-rays over many years may possibly contribute to the development of cancer.

My doctor had told me that I had fibrocystic breasts and that lumpiness was characteristic of this condition. I told her that I thought fibrocystic disease was a misnomer because to my knowledge half of all women had fibrocystic breasts and it was no big deal. Actually, I was unaware that my breasts were lumpy; even though I checked them for lumps fairly regularly, the only breasts I had ever felt were my own, and they felt normal to me.

When I arranged for my annual checkup around the time of my forty-third birthday, I was a little concerned. I had felt an obvious lump the size of a large marble in my left breast. When the doctor examined the lump, she said it was a good sign that the lump was movable. This time when she recommended a mammogram I agreed without arguing. She called me the next day with the results: the lump did not show up on the mammogram, but a few dots of calcification elsewhere in the breast did. She explained that these dots (like grains of sand) were indicative of cancer and urged me to make an appointment with the surgeon to determine whether a biopsy was needed.

The surgeon recommended that I have the lump and the area where the calcification dots had shown up on the mammogram both biopsied. He recommended that I have this done as outpatient surgery under general anesthesia. I scheduled the biopsy for a few weeks later. This gave me time to attend to some out-of-town business and to do some study about breast cancer. I read about various types of biopsies in the medical literature and learned that needle biopsies that could be done easily in a doctor's office were not 100-percent conclusive. Because there was a strong possibility of cancer in another part of my breast as well as in the lump I had found, I decided that surgical excision of the lump for biopsy was a good idea. Not only would I be rid of the lump but I'd have the most accurate diagnosis of its nature.

Prior to the biopsy, I was sent to the medical director of my HMO who had to approve all outpatient surgery. By that time I had read enough to ask a dozen questions, few of which he was able to answer. He signed the necessary papers approving the biopsy, and I was admitted to day surgery two days after my forty-third birthday.

The lump in my breast was obvious to the surgeon, but the area where there were a few microscopic dots was not. He sent me back to mammography so that dots could be localized. This was done by inserting a needle into the breast and taking mammograms (eight) until the needle could be seen in the affected area. Then a small amount of blue dye was injected to make the area visible. Although other women have told me it was a terrible experience for them, this procedure caused me little discomfort. I think the reason I tolerated it so well is that my primary doctor had explained the procedure to me, and I was anticipating it. The other women had not been warned that this procedure might be necessary.

Before falling asleep with intravenous Valium, I told the surgeon I wanted an estrogen assay test done. Rose Kushner had recommended this in her book *Alternatives*,* in which she describes her battle with breast cancer. The surgeon assured me that the assay test would be done if there was enough tissue to do it. He and my own doctor had both informed me that the test required a fairly large amount of cancerous tissue and that I probably would not have enough.

At noon, I was discharged from day surgery with the welcome news that the frozen section revealed my condition to be benign. The lump had been a harmless cyst. I was instructed to return to the surgeon in a week to have my stitches removed. I spent the rest of the day in bed at home. I was groggy from the anesthesia and very grateful to my sweetheart, Paul, who accompanied me to surgery, made me chicken soup, and assured me of his love regardless of the outcome. I had decided not to worry about possible results of the permanent section, which would be more accurate than the frozen section in diagnosing cancer but would take a few days for the results to be known.

The next day the surgeon called to ask how I was. Although I assured him that I had changed my own dressing and that the incisions looked fine, he asked me to come to his office the next day. When I arrived, he told me that the permanent section had revealed cancer. The lump was indeed a harmless cyst, but there was cancer in the area where the little dots were. He urged me to have a mastectomy (modified radical) and said he was also obligated to inform me that I might choose radiation as an alternative form of therapy. He believed mastectomy was preferable and urged me to have it very soon as tumors sometimes grow more quickly after biopsy

---

* Kushner, Rose, *Alternatives* (Cambridge, MA: The Kensington Press, 1984).

(not true, I read later). He also warned me about the doubling time of tumors and warned me to not waste a lot of time making a decision.

This was a big blow. Instead of heading for the liquor cabinet, I decided to waste no time learning as much as I could about various treatments for breast cancer. I made up my mind that, although I wanted advice from various medical specialists, no one but me would decide what course of action I would take. The first place I looked for information was my own medical library, which had scarce information. The best article I had was a summary of the Fisher report comparing mastectomies with lumpectomies and radiation in the National Women's Health Network newsletter.* A more complete report of Fisher's work had been published in the *New England Journal of Medicine*,** and my mother, who worked as a hospital volunteer, photocopied what I wanted at the hospital's medical library. The public library had some old books about breast cancer, none of which was particularly helpful. The local feminist bookstore had several good books (including Rose Kushner's). A trip to the Women's Health Exchange at the University of Illinois provided more helpful information. I had heard about the Women's Health Exchange from some of my friends in Cassandra, the radical feminist nurses network; one of them also gave me an old copy of *The Breast Cancer Digest* and suggested I contact Y-Me, a support group for women with breast cancer. None of these resources had much information

---

* National Women's Health Network, 1325 G St. NW, Washington, DC 20005

** Fisher, Bernard, M.D., "Ten-Year Results of a Randomized Clinical Trial Comparing Radical Mastectomy and Total Mastectomy with or without Radiation," *New England Journal of Medicine*, 321:11 (March 14, 1985), pp. 674–681.

about microscopic cancers. Almost everything I read talked about solid tumors.

I called the National Cancer Institute to see whether they had a more current edition of *The Breast Cancer Digest*; they agreed to send me a copy, and it turned out to be a goldmine of information. The book contained summaries of many of the articles I had spent hours looking up in medical libraries. I also called the American Cancer Society Information Service. The w

oman who handled my call recommended that I ask the surgeon for a copy of the pathologist's report rather than rely on a few notes I had taken when I spoke with the surgeon on the phone.

When I went to the surgeon's office to pick up the report, he again urged me to have a mastectomy without undue delay. He kept referring to my tumor, although the pathologist's report referred only to a few abnormal cells that had been removed in the biopsy. The pathologist had written that the specimen from the first incision was a cyst and that I had fibrocystic disease. The specimen from the second incision where the dots had been showed a few dilated ducts filled with abnormal proliferating duct cells. Her conclusion was "fibrocystic disease of breast with focal intraductal carcinoma."

The surgeon annoyed me with his repeated use of the word *tumor*. The way I saw it, the cells had not yet formed a tumor and the cancerous area had been removed in the biopsy. He said that if I decided to have radiation instead of a mastectomy that he would need to do a quadrantectomy first. Again he warned me about doubling time and urged me to make a decision soon. My reading had taught me that doubling time ranged from about 20 days to 210 days. That seemed to give me plenty of time in the event cancerous cells remained in my breast. From the way the surgeon talked, one would think cancer cells doubled every five minutes. He resented some of my questions and discouraged discussion if I disagreed with him. I went home feeling angry and upset, feelings I experienced frequently over the subsequent few weeks. Intellectually I could deal with the situation and was not surprised at any of the answers or attitudes people presented to me, but—as one of my friends explained—it's one thing to understand something in your head and quite another for your gut to deal with it.

My stitches were removed on the ninth day after the biopsy, and I took off for Ann Arbor, Michigan, for the continental Cassandra gathering. My nurse practitioner friend Elizabeth drove up with me. She warned me not to jump into radical treatment unless I was convinced of its necessity. As we drove, she described several instances of unnecessary medical or surgical intervention to me. At the gathering, I announced my medical problem to the nurses present and asked for anyone with some knowledge about breast cancer to talk with me. A few of them referred me to nurse friends who were doing research on breast cancer. One said that both her mother and grandmother had died of breast cancer and that she was at high risk to get it. She advised me to get a second pathologist's report as well as second opinions on treatment and urged me to take the time I needed to make an intelligent decision on treatment.

When I returned home, I read more about the Fisher study that had made headlines a few months previously. Dr. Bernard Fisher had concluded that whether women have a mastectomy or a lumpectomy or a lumpectomy and radiation, survival rates were about the same over a five-year period. I was anxious to begin discussing treatment options with my internist. She was on vacation, so I saw my old doctor who amused me with his coffee cup stating "accurate guesswork done here." He did not know a lot about breast cancer, but he thought I should consider radiation. He urged me to talk to the cancer specialist at the HMO. When my internist returned from vacation, I saw her; she urged me to have a mastectomy and told me horror stories of people who had radiation.

The next day I saw the oncologist. He was far more knowledgeable than the internists and answered my questions accurately and appropriately. He agreed that there was no single best method to handle my cancer. We discussed risk factors, statistics, and other issues. He recommended that I have a lymph node biopsy. I was still sore from the first biopsy and did not want another unless it was necessary.

My next consultation was with the radiologist. He shocked me. He told me he did not believe in radiation as primary therapy for breast cancer. He told me my cancer was too minor for radiation and that I should have a mastectomy. He charged my HMO $100 for this consultation. At that point more than ever before, I was struck by the difference between medical research findings and what is actually practiced in the medical community.

I wanted another medical opinion. A woman at the Y-Me office referred me to the comprehensive breast center at Rush-Presbyterian-St. Luke's Medical Center. The program there sounded promising, so I arranged an appointment at my own expense and brought my pathology slides and mammograms. It was important to me that I be able to speak with the three specialists I would see there (surgeon, radiologist, oncologist) at the same time. If they disagreed with one another, I wanted them to discuss troublesome issues with each other and me at the same time.*

This pathologist had a different diagnosis: lobular cancer in situ. This diagnosis meant that it could be years before the cancer would recur and that it could recur in either breast. The chances of lymph node involvement were estimated at one percent.

With this diagnosis, I decided that I would go for medical follow-up on a regular basis but that was all. The breast team said that mastectomy or radiation therapy would be the safest route for me to go but that it would not be unreasonable for me to go for breast checkups every three months and mammograms every year (more often if indicated). With only a one-percent chance of lymph node involvement, biopsy to check my lymph nodes hardly seemed worthwhile. I promised myself I would examine my breasts regularly and keep myself informed about new developments in the diagnosis and treatment of breast cancer.

Having made that decision, I felt greatly relieved and wanted to get on with my life. All was well. Once again, I began to feel invincible. I saw my doctor every year and went for mammograms that were negative. At an examination two years later, my internist felt uncomfortable about the hard lumpiness in my left breast. She said it might be my fibrocystic condition but that I should think about going back to the comprehensive breast center to see whether the specialists there thought I should have a biopsy even though my latest mammogram was negative also. I arranged an appointment and took my

---

* A friend in Cassandra suggested that I would get more out of the discussion if I could listen to it later when my anxiety level was lower, so I got the doctors to agree to have me make an audiotape of the meeting.

mammograms with me. The surgeon agreed the mammograms were negative; he told me that the chance of the lumpiness being malignant was only ten to twenty percent. I decided that this risk was too great not to do something, so I arranged for a biopsy through my HMO. Again I went to day surgery; this time when I woke from the anesthesia I was informed that I had a malignancy.

I named my left breast Bernadette Arnold because I felt betrayed—and I scheduled a mastectomy as soon as possible. The surgery went well, and losing my breast did not bother me nearly as much as I thought it would. My friends, family, and colleagues sent cards and flowers that filled the room. I looked forward to going home and returning to work, secure in the knowledge that with a modified radical mastectomy I would quickly regain the full use of my left arm and that Paul would love me with or without a breast.

On my second postoperative day, an internist came to my room with news: cancer had been found in ten lymph nodes. I couldn't believe it. I panicked. For the first time, I truly felt that my life was being threatened. The internist spent several minutes with me until I calmed down and assured me that I did not have to handle phone calls and visitors if I didn't feel like it. I called Paul; he came over and held my hand and told me he was with me. Later that day, the oncologist came to see me. He told me that my cancer was hormone-dependent for both estrogen and progesterone and that he would start me on tamoxifen to block the effects of estrogen and then chemotherapy to destroy any remaining cancer cells.

My anxiety level was extremely high. As a nurse, my experiences with chemotherapy were limited to terminally ill patients who were treated in a research project in a university hospital twenty-five years ago and whose death was sometimes hastened by the toxic effects of the chemicals. I was afraid that the side effects of chemotherapy would make me sick and unable to work, and the possibility of losing my independence filled me with dread.

A few days later I was discharged form the hospital, and I applied for a sick leave at work. The oncologist assured me I would probably be able to continue working during the six months I would receive chemotherapy, but I didn't know whether to believe him. I arrived home in my panicky state and tried to get a handle on my anxiety.

My daughter was a young adult who ordinarily spent more time away from our apartment than she did in it; she made a point of spending more time with me. Just being with her and feeling the love we shared meant a great deal to me. Some of the school nurses, professional colleagues of mine, who had come to see me at the hospital came to see me at home. They brought homemade casseroles and books on nutrition, and I was extremely touched by their thoughtfulness and caring. One had a friend who had had a recent mastectomy, and she told me where to go for a customized prosthesis and bras.*

I received eight chemotherapy treatments over a six-month period. My first one was scheduled just a few weeks after surgery. It turned out to be quite tolerable—nothing like that experience I had dreaded. The nurses who started the IV and administered the powerful drugs warned me that I would lose my hair very soon and recommended that I get a wig before the next treatment. They suggested that I get

---

* Although some feminists have refused to wear a prosthesis, I wanted one so I could feel normal when I put on my clothes. I had no interest whatsoever in surgery to reconstruct a breast.

a good one and told me of some places where patients had been most satisfied. Following their advice, I bought a good, custom-made wig that looked natural (except that it always looked good). It seemed expensive, but the cost was no more than what I would have spent on haircuts and perma- nents during the year I wore it. Shortly after my first chemotherapy treatment I returned to work.

Support from friends and family meant a lot to me during this difficult time. My father accompa- nied me to the chemotherapy treatments, and my parents insisted on taking me out to dinner every few weeks. My friends kept in close touch with me, calling and sending cards and encouragement. I went to Y-Me support group meetings for a while because I was aware that I needed to talk with women who had overcome their anxieties in dealing with cancer and were able to do what they had to do to continue living successfully. Before long I felt that I was giving more support that I was getting, and I stopped going.

The most striking thing about this time was that I no longer had any desire to learn or read anything about breast cancer. If I came across an article in the newspaper, I would force myself to read it, but every feature inevitably started out with statistics of women who were dying from this disease. I would be depressed and restless for days after reading an article or seeing anything about breast cancer on tele- vision. This was dramatically different from the preceding two years during which I had been relent- less in seeking information about breast cancer. Armed with all that knowledge, I had made a deci- sion I later believed had been wrong. My cancer had spread as a result of my decision. I had a mental block to new information; that block lasted a couple of years.

During this time, I wished I had a church to turn to for solace. Like other disillusioned women, I had lost hope that the Catholic Church would ever recognize that women have a right to equality and reproductive rights, and I no longer considered myself part of the Church. I asked a friend who had attended divinity school for some pastoral counseling. At her suggestion, I bought a book of Psalms written in inclusive language to help me meditate. A few days later I picked up a copy of *Letting God: Christian Meditations for Recovering Persons.* The title appealed to me because I liked to think of myself as a recovering person rather than a cancer victim. Several days into my reading of the book, it dawned on my that the book was written for alcoholics. The book filled me with hope, and I read each day's meditation for a year and a half.

Life and relationships with family and friends have become precious to me. I bought a house shortly after completing chemotherapy and married Paul a year later. I try harder now to keep in contact with my nurse friends. In my work as a school nurse, I am now better able to provide support to students with cancer and other serious diseases. I am able to be a better friend to other women who have cancer. I'm a little heavier than I used to be; part of the reason is that I don't want to waste away too soon if my cancer should spread.

A cornerstone of the women's movement is the belief that "the personal is political"; I am trying to muster the energy to fight cancer as a political issue. A high fat diet has been implicated in breast cancer, and I volunteered for a research project designed to see whether a low-fat diet would help reduce breast cancer in women. The project was canceled before it got off the ground. Rose Kushner started a political action committee (PAC) for breast cancer; I sent her a check and a note, hoping she would tell me what else I could do, but I got no response.

Congresswoman Rose Marie Oakar says that we should be very angry about the fact that so many women are getting cancer. She says we should demand that our government put more money and effort into preventing breast cancer and finding cures. When my union has its blood drive and mini health fair next year, we will have at least investigated the possibility of having a mobile unit that provides mammograms there. And when we hold a women's rights conference in March, one of the workshops will be on women's health issues. I'm starting to clip articles about women's groups or individuals who are doing something politically to fight cancer and believe that this will be a growing movement. A tremendous amount of money is now going for research and services related to AIDS. People concerned about AIDS have mobilized into a powerful lobbying group. People concerned about cancer need to do the same.

My initial experience with cancer showed me that there is a big gap between medical research and medical practice. My second experience showed me how vulnerable human beings, including me, are to life-threatening illness. As a feminist, I am always working on some project or other—reproductive rights, family leave, equal opportunity. I feel that I ought to be actively trying to get this country committed to the elimination of breast cancer, ovarian cancer, and other diseases of women, yet my energy for this is rather low at this time. My own wounds are still too fresh for me to charge into battle. But as women begin to speak out and move into action, our collective energy will increase and we can hope that our daughters will not have to live with the same fear of cancer we have faced.

Lesbians Evolving Health Care:
Our Lives Depend on It*

Jackie Winnow

Recently the *San Francisco Chronicle* ran an article addressing the plight of the hundred women with AIDS in the Bay Area and describing the services that have been started for them, including housing, childcare, a day center, haircutting, a food bank, massage, counseling and meals.

In 1988, approximately forty thousand women were living with cancer in the San Francisco/Oakland area, at least four thousand being lesbians, about four thousand women dying. Eight thousand women were diagnosed this year. The forty thousand women don't have the services that the hundred women with AIDS have. I want the women with AIDS to have those services. I don't mean to polarize. But I also want recognition that we have a huge problem here and we need to do something about it.

According to the American Cancer Society, half a million women in the United States will be diagnosed with cancer in 1989, and a quarter million will die from the disease. Forty-two thousand women will die from breast cancer in one year, about the same number of people who have died in the first

---

* This article was adapted and shortened from the keynote speech at the Lesbian Caregivers & the AIDS Epidemic Conference in San Francisco in January 1989; and is an edited version of the same paper published in *Out/Look* No. 5, summer 1989, entitled "Lesbians Working on AIDS: Assessing the Impact on Health Care for Women." It was published in this version in *Sinister Wisdom 39: On Disability* (winter 1989–90).

23

ten years of the AIDS epidemic. Cancer is the lead-
ing cause of death in women ages 35 to 54. Cancer
has become an acceptable epidemic. As someone
who has metastatic breast cancer, that is unacceptable to me.

While many lesbians continued to keep their attention primarily focused on women and women's
concerns, many more women turned toward AIDS
work, as shown by our numbers at this conference.

Why have so many of us become AIDS caregivers? There is a clear, delineated crisis and there is
a need to help people in our community. We take
care of our friends who need us. Because women,
even lesbians, were raised to be caregivers, we
moved toward that need. We were raised to despise
ourselves and belittle our needs while holding those
of men to be important. Women were raised to take
care of men and to serve them. My father once told
me that.

And even though we are lesbians and have made
conscious choices to disown that heritage, we have
nonetheless incorporated many of its basic tenets. As
the "other" in the lesbian and gay and women's
movements, we were left out a lot, not part of the in-
crowd. Working in AIDS, coming to the service of
men—working in their agenda finally—served to
validate our existence. It is also easier to work on
something like AIDS, because, by and large, we
won't get AIDS, nor will our lovers or our lesbian
neighbors. And AIDS is something the whole society
is addressing; we can actually fit in, we can be considered heroic and important and decent and be
recognized for it. We can even, sometimes, work in a
queer environment. We get to work where our
hearts lie. The work structures are set out for us; the
funding is available.

This is not to say that working on AIDS is easy or that we don't care for and love the people we know with AIDS. It is to say that we make excruciating choices without even being aware of them.

Lesbians were and still are in the vanguard of the women's and lesbian and gay liberation movements. Without us, there would be no rape crisis centers, no women's foundations or buildings, no awareness of domestic violence, no women's music festivals or women's radio programming. There would be no National March on Washington, AIDS quilts, AIDS food banks or many other AIDS services, especially those for women. Without us, the women's movement would not have addressed homophobia and heterosexism and the lesbian/gay movement would not have addressed sexism. Indeed, without us, these movements would have remained one-dimensional reform movements. With us, they become dynamic forces for social change.

What has happened to the women's movement and community since the AIDS crisis started? While it still pulses with creativity and excitement, many institutions, organizations, services and political agenda have been slowed or disappeared. Not just because of AIDS, but because of general disinterest. Here in the Bay Area, there is no more *Plexus*, A Woman's Place Bookstore, Berkeley Women's Center, San Francisco Women's Health Center or Lilith Theater group, to name just a few.

Right-wing groups like Operation Rescue are harassing women at abortion and birth control clinics and bombing those clinics. Why aren't we marching in large numbers to protest? Violence against women is proliferating at enormous rates; we're murdered, raped and beaten every few seconds, yet few people decry violence against women. Why don't we make it clear that there is a hate cam-

paign targeting women and that it is not new? Why
aren't we screaming that sexism kills?

No one takes care of women or lesbians except
women or lesbians, and we have a hard time taking
care of ourselves, of finding ourselves worthy and
important enough to pay attention to. Why don't we
even consider our needs urgent?

▲ ▲ ▲

As a woman with cancer, I have learned about
how serious our needs are, about what we need and
what we don't have. As Lesbian/Gay Liaison to the
San Francisco Human Rights Commission, I found
myself waiting for my first biopsy results in May of
1985 at a Lesbian/Gay Advisory Committee meeting. Our meetings focused on AIDS and I remember
thinking, screaming internally really, "What about
me?" Well, I quickly found out what about me.

I felt invisible in our community. I had a lumpectomy followed by radiation, survived, and was
expected to go back to work—to work on AIDS—
and life. There was little recognition of what a
woman with cancer goes through. What I found was
a community willing to address AIDS, but no more.
I found that the things that were offered for people
with AIDS did not exist for people with other life-
threatening illnesses; that some of the problems that
existed for people with AIDS existed for all people
with life-threatening illnesses, and yet our community, and society in general, has been
one-dimensional in its approach.

If you have AIDS in San Francisco, you can go to
the AIDS Foundation for food and social services
advocacy, get emergency funding through the AIDS
Emergency Fund, and get excellent meals through
Project Open Hand. Your pets are taken care of if

you should land in the hospital or if you're too sick to take care of them. There are clinics and alternative centers and organizations fighting for drugs, research and mental health.

If you have cancer, you wait endlessly for a support group, which if you are a lesbian, a woman of color, working class, or believe in alternatives, you don't fit into anyway. No organization shepherds you through the social service maze, no organization brings you luscious meals or sends support people to clean your house or hold your hand. No organization fights for your needs; no one advocates for you.

I'm not saying this just to pick on our community. We live in a society that, by and large, does not take care of its sick. In the case of AIDS, we have built a model as a community. This model does not exist outside of AIDS. This model was built by lesbians and gay men to serve people with AIDS, but it does not serve our entire community.

Cancer, like AIDS, is about living; it's about living with a life-threatening disease, in whatever stage, whatever condition. Although each of us experiences cancer individually, it is through collective support and action that changes take place. As an activist, I always believed that, and my own cancer experience strengthened that belief even more.

Organizing is needed for all diseases. All disease and illness in this country is political, not just AIDS. For myself, I learned to make a will, a durable power of attorney, to have someone at doctor's visits, to tape-record those visits, to build support.

And I took some of what I learned doing AIDS work and a lot of what I learned from feminist organizing and women's liberation, and with other women, created the Women's Cancer Resource Center. We desperately needed a resource, support and advocacy center where women with cancer could be

empowered to make their own choices and be sup-
ported by other women in their situation, a center
controlled by women with cancer.

The Women's Cancer Resource Center has been
slow to grow, partly because some of us had or have
cancer and need to take care of our health. Additionally, a lot of energy is going into AIDS from the
women's community, and there is little left over for
cancer or other disease and disabilities. Regardless
of AIDS, women have reduced their organizing
work and settled into solely working on themselves
instead.

Although we are an agency that serves all women
with cancer, we are not in the closet about having lesbians on the advisory committee or serving lesbians.
Consequently, we receive little funding due to homophobia. Funding agencies think they are funding the
gay community through AIDS. Women's groups controlled by women and for women get little funding
by foundations, businesses, people with money, gay
men, or other women. Women's agencies are not so
popular; women's issues get pushed aside.

Despite all those obstacles, the Women's Cancer
Resource Center thrives. We've just gotten our own
space. The advisory committee works on funding
and programming; we have support groups; we do
forums and educationals, and information and refer-
ral and counseling and speak out about the politics
of cancer.

▲ ▲ ▲

When I found another lump in the same breast, I
went for further tests and discovered that the cancer
had spread to my lungs and bones. I could not
believe that I was so ill. I had been exercising, feeling great, working long hours, just like the first time.

I knew the implications; I knew women who had died of metastatic breast cancer. Yet, the reality is also one of survival—and for a good and productive life. It is now more than a year later. In my first round with cancer, I was always making decisions that had to do with my survival; this time, I agonized over every decision as my life lay fragilely before me.

I made my decisions with what I had learned as a cancer and AIDS activist, as a feminist. I went through my treatments, I did my research, and live with a great deal of support from my lover Teya and my friends and acquaintances. With the first diagnosis, my life's axis permanently tilted; with this diagnosis, I live constantly on the edge.

From this vantage point, there are certain things I want you to know, to take with you, to think about, to change.

The most important thing I want you to know is that lesbians do not have a support network. Disabled women have found it ironic that this conference is addressing lesbian caregivers in relation to the AIDS service community, but not the women's community. One woman told me that although about 80 percent of the disability attendants used to be lesbians, there are only a handful left.

Support and caregiving in the lesbian community often becomes a matter of personality. There are so many women with health problems, be they cancer, environmental illness, chronic immune deficiency syndrome (Epstein Barr), multiple sclerosis—but no one recognizes that these are serious illnesses, and that they need to be taken care of. Indeed, because they are women, the community has not mobilized.

Just as we were healers, experts in our fields in the Middle Ages, we need to lay claim to our heri-

tage now. We have many people in nascent stages of
expertise, but few experts. When we started the
women's health movement, we were taking control
of our bodies, mostly in the areas of reproductive
and gynecological health care. Now we need experts
in cancer, lupus, arthritis, environmental illness. I
mean practitioners in allopathic medicine, Chinese
medicine, or homeopathy. Going to a doctor, hoping
for non-homophobia, is not enough. We need practitioners and clinics that are supportive of us as
lesbians and experts in their fields.

When lesbians get sick, they also get poor. Women
are on the lower rung of the financial ladder, and
when they become ill, the bottom falls out much
quicker because they are closer to it. They lose their
health insurance and can't get any anymore. If they
are lucky enough to have a job, they have to stay in
it. Many women I know work when the act of working is almost physically unbearable because they
can't afford anything else. Some women would love
to work but no one will hire them. Some women are
on SSI but hardly making it since, cruelly, the
amount is so low.

AIDS is a new disease and fresh in terms of who
controls information about it. Information and
resources about cancer, however, historically have
been controlled by the American Cancer Society. Its
board, as well as those of other cancer institutions, is
composed of people with a lot of power to keep
things as they are: chemical company executives, the
Rockefellers, the very scientists standing to get
money. Research is geared toward big bucks, not to
actual prevention.

Actual prevention would mean changing society—
cleaning it up—and that won't happen. When they
say prevention, they quite often are talking about
small individual prevention like quitting smoking

and cutting fat consumption, or early detection, like mammograms or self-breast exams. When they find a tumor in your breast in a mammogram, you already have cancer. They don't mean going after the tobacco industry; they don't mean stopping pollution or providing quality food.

We need a National Cancer Institute that does relevant research—not research into a quick cure that costs a fortune, but into real prevention, into real cure. Everyone know pollution causes cancer, but does NCI or the American Cancer Society do anything about it?

That's where AIDS can make some inroads. Just like we question what is said about AIDS, we need to question what is said about cancer or chronic fatigue immune deficiency, or any other disease. We need to question current concepts of disease.

There are a few things going on in society, in which our community participates, that I find particularly obnoxious. Over the past several years, the women's movement had become coopted by professionalism. This has also happened in the world around us. Our society has taken the individual who may have known something and rendered that person useless, so that she has to turn toward experts to tell her what to do. What they usually tell her is individualizing and internalizing.

Earlier in the women's movement we took what victimized us—rape, battery, incest—and worked toward changing society, while making ourselves stronger. Now we work on ourselves individually. Most of the work is therapy work. Without changing the environment which allows such victimization to take place, it is allowed to continue. In that vein, there is a new disease model which holds the individual responsible for her illness. I call it dumping. I call it psychobabble.

With it has come a lot of new-age jargon about the
fitness of self. We are a culture obsessed with what
the individual can do to look good and stay
healthy—we can jog, exercise, eat oat bran, stop
smoking. This is not to say that people cannot affect
their own health. But this form of thinking says that
it is all in our power. So if we don't stay healthy, we
must have done something, or worse yet, if she
doesn't stay healthy, she must have done something.
It doesn't change a thing; it internalizes illness and
blames the victim.

This form of thinking plays out the concept that
we create our own reality, that we have ultimate freedom of choice and total control. Fuck the world
around us, the people around us, the government
and corporations, even our own biology. They don't
exist. They don't affect us. There are no such things
as sexism, homophobia, racism, anti-Semitism, capitalism, pollution, biology.

I cannot begin to tell you the number of people
who believe and have said that I must not have had
a positive attitude, or I wouldn't have gotten cancer.
This is cruel. People say, don't get angry, anger is
bad. I have heard that I worked too hard, that if I
had just concentrated on myself I wouldn't have gotten sick. Don't do anything meaningful. This
thinking comes from a society that doesn't want us
to be angry, that doesn't want us to be activists.

Some people say having cancer is a gift. Having a
life-threatening illness is not a gift. You wouldn't
want me to give you cancer and I don't want it
either. Yes, my life has changed, and yes, I have
learned from the experience. But I don't have cancer
because I have something to learn from it. I have
cancer because the cells in my body malfunctioned.

Cancer is said to be an emotionally caused disease
because the scientists don't have a cure for it and

they are not sure how it is caused. If we keep it on an individual level, we need never find that cause or the cure. Before they found a cure for tuberculosis, TB was thought to be emotionally based. There was a TB personality just like there is a cancer personality, and people tried to visualize away their illness. As Susan Sontag described in *Illness as Metaphor*, once a cure was found for TB, all that was tossed out.

The other dangerous thing we have in our community is the idea that not only do emotions cause cancer, spirituality does too. Somehow something we have done in the past is causing our troubles now; we are working out our karma, what goes around comes around. I guess that's why women are raped and Black people are lynched—it's karma. Take the onus off the perpetrator. Accept the unacceptable. Forgive the unforgivable.

Somehow a community founded on feminist principles, a community founded to change society and its structures to those that are life-affirming, has taken on the individualist ideals of capitalism. By doing this, we unthinkingly tossed out the notion that we are impacted by our society and our deeds affect that society. Until we understand that our actions are meaningful, we will work individually and change will not occur.

I think this has happened partly because it is easier to deal with disease, or any wrong, really, on an individual basis. That way we can believe it won't happen to us and we can maintain the illusion that we have control in a society out of control.

We live in a world with acid rain, with a hole in the ozone layer, where food is mass produced and picked early with no nutrients, where pesticides are sprayed on the workers and the food we eat, where the animals we eat are raised in a tortured environment and fed hormones and antibiotics; we live in a world that has chemical dumps under housing tracts, schools, playgrounds, with nuclear weapons and dumps, where winds spread radiation over all of us. This is labelled pollution when, in fact, it is invisible violence.

Our country has no national health care system. Society turns away from the homeless. Chemical company executives sit on the boards of the largest cancer organizations and control what kind of research is done. Society must change and redirect itself to be life-affirming; where individual welfare and health care is respected; where profits don't count more than people; where we are free of chemical and radiation hazards; where good healthy food is available; where each person is known to be significant and worthy of life.

Let's see ourselves as healers, as workers. We need to make connections and engage in critical thinking, to see the universality and interconnectedness of issues. We need to take the skills we have learned as feminists and apply them to our work on AIDS and to our work with women. And then take the skills we have from working with AIDS and apply them to working in women's health care. Let's bring it back home.

As individuals in partnership with others, we have to be working on women's health issues. We can strongly protest a Department of Public Health for not funding women-specific health care. We can be out there in huge numbers protecting reproductive health and fighting the Operation Rescue people. We can build a lesbian-health support network, so that lesbians who need help are brought meals, taken to appointments and so on. We can support institutions like the Women's Cancer Resource Center financially and through our skills. We can do this and more. We need to be screaming in the streets that we will not be killed by the dissolution of the earth and make the government accountable to the people.

I have wondered whether the urgency I feel comes because I have cancer, but I think that it only has brought it closer to me. I firmly believe that we are on the brink and that we must be very forceful in order to stop the destruction before there is no us. We have to stop being nice girls, and start fighting as if our live depend on it because they do.

Special acknowledgment and thanks to my lover Teya Schaffer.

No Big Deal

Jane Murtaugh

"No big deal," my doctor said as he reported the results of my pap smear. "No big deal, these things are often wrong." Thus began my six-year struggle with various forms of cancer. I had gone in for the first pap smear of my life in January 1975 and the results had been a "3," which means that there is a high probability of cervical cancer. The test was to be repeated by a specialist in obstetrics and gynecology the next week.

When I went in for the second test, the doctor reported that he thought he could see an abnormality in the cells of my cervix. When the smear results came back they were different. This time they showed clearly that I did have cancer of the cervix, a fairly uncommon occurance in girls nineteen years of age. I visited a gynecological oncologist who informed me, after reading my test results, that he believed that this form of cancer was treatable with chemotherapy but that few patients lived longer that two years. He suggested that we start on a serious regimen of new anti-cancer antibiotics immediately.

After a great deal of panic and some real soul searching, I decided that I did not want to live the last years of my life taking medication to extend my life and at the same time make it a misery. I did not agree to the chemotherapy.

I was advised to get a second opinion. I asked for the name of another doctor, made an appointment, had a uterine and cervical biopsy, and was told something completely different: According to this doctor, what I had was not a serious form of cervical cancer and could be treated with a series of radiation treatments that should begin as soon as possible.

Radiation was an experience. These treatments consisted of inserting a metal rod through my vagina and up to my cervix. The rod was connected to a cobalt machine that gave me the necessary radiation. The procedure was somewhat painful; more difficult was the indignity of it, and I would not allow anyone else to accompany me for the treatment. It was many years before I could tell anyone about what these treatments were like.

As a student at a small college in Indiana, I expected support from fellow students and staff. But since my hair did not fall out and I did not lose vast amounts of weight (in fact, because I suffered edema as a side effect, I seemed to gain weight), most people got very tired of hearing of my fears and sad stories.

I did not tell my parents that I had cancer because I knew my mother would want to bring me home and take care of me. I felt as though that would be giving in to the disease. I tried to pretend that everything was normal, that I was not ill, and that everything would be O.K. I became depressed and rather angry.

The cancer responded well to radiation and, although it recurred almost immediately, treatment as prescribed seemed to take care of the problem. After nearly two years of treatment (once for the original lesion, and later when it recurred) I found myself in the limbo of the newly cured, in which many people find themselves counting the days, weeks, and so on until they can consider themselves "safe."

But I would never be the same. I had a sample of how it felt to be "terminal," if only for a few days. I had also become aware of how it is to have cancer and to be perceived by both teachers and peers as an untouchable. Friends grew tired of listening and were unable be supportive. My grades went down as faculty members grew tired of hearing about my "health problems" when assignments came in late, or when I missed classes because I was ill from radiation therapy.

It wasn't just that I was unable to carry my full load. I represented the fear that many people seem to carry with them. Most informed people realize that cancer is not spread through physical contact, but fear is not rational. And fear of cancer is real.

Time went on, and my pap smears and biopsies were fine. This reprieve ended my senior year of college, when I had a menstrual period that did not stop. After three months of bleeding (which I tried to ignore) I started hemorrhaging and I found myself hospitalized for anemia and to have a D&C (dilation and curettage). Because my blood count was so low, the doctors chose to do a uterine biopsy instead; it was fine. No sign of cancer. I graduated from college and immediately began teaching Special Education in a small town called Hope.

But I was gaining weight. I had always been overweight, but my weight was clearly out of control. I tried dieting over the summer, but my weight kept going up and up. Then on Labor Day weekend 1978, I became ill with what I thought was a severe case of intestinal flu. I could not eat or drink. I was in severe abdominal distress and could not move without great pain. I missed the first week of school and forced myself to go back after that by convincing myself I felt better.

In the meantime I went to the doctor. He gave me some antibiotics to clear up what he thought was a secondary infection and sent me home to lose weight.

If I had learned anything from my first bout with cancer, it was to find a different doctor if I couldn't believe what one had to say. I knew that I was continuing to gain weight and that I was barely eating. I was in real pain. And I discovered was that doctors discounted what I was saying almost completely. They clearly thought that my problem was obesity and hysteria. In their favor, I will say that I had every x-ray there was to be had and every medication, especially antibiotics, that could be prescribed. Nothing helped.

But I knew there was something very wrong. I looked pregnant, weighed 431 pounds, and measured 72 inches around my waist. I could barely walk and breathing was painful. I had refused even the mention of surgery, but finally, after the fourth doctor I saw suggested that I might be having gall bladder pain, I acquiesced and visited a surgeon in my hometown.

The surgeon agreed that I probably had gall stones; surgery was scheduled for two weeks hence. The doctor was planning a working trip to Haiti and I needed time to settle affairs at home before moving in with my parents to recover.

As it happened, my sister had to come and rescue me.

I woke up one morning and was unable to move. My sister came to my apartment, got me down the stairs and into her car, and took me to my parents' house. I stayed there until the day arrived for me to enter the hospital. My mom is a nurse and took very good care of me. While I stayed at my parents' house, I felt better than I had in months; it was a relief to let myself relax. But I remember entering the hospital after that week with my parents. I felt like I would never be able to leave. I thought I was going to die.

Terror is the word that comes to mind when I think of that time in my life. I could not move and I was sure this was cancer. I thought that when they performed surgery, they would open me up and close me back because there would be nothing they could do.

And then there were the tests. All the tests all of the other doctors had done had been reordered for this week, though I had brought the x-rays and lab reports with me. I was completely miserable. I was not in control of my own body, my own life. The hospital staff, while caring and empathetic, felt the need to follow my doctor's orders to the letter. And he was in Haiti. I did not see a doctor for the six days I was in the hospital before he returned.

But I learned something. I learned that I could say "No!" and that tests would not be run. I learned that they do not boil patients in oil for refusing to take one more laxative as a prep for one more test. In fact I felt their relief at my refusal. It could be my fault when the good doctor returned and the tests were not done.

And there was a scene when the doctor returned, but I won that shouting match. He did not realize he had the previous test results and films. He did not understand how much pain I was in. I even feel that I gained his respect, a lesson I will long remember.

Surgery was performed as scheduled. But instead of a 45-minute cholecystectomy (gall bladder removal), surgery lasted four and one half hours. They found a 47-pound ovarian cyst with a bag attached containing five gallons of fluid. While trying to remove the cyst, the doctors also found it necessary to remove my gall bladder (which did contain stones), my right ovary, eighteen inches of my small intestine, part of my liver, my spleen, and of course my appendix. It made the local news. I lost more than 80 pounds on the table and would lose another 100 pounds over the course of the next few months.

Through the initial period of recovery from surgery, I was immediately relieved of pain. I did request pain medication occasionally, but I took it because I was afraid, not in pain. And for almost six days, I was heady with relief.

That was not to last. Recovery from abdominal surgery is not easy. And I was told that while the tumor was not malignant, the fluid was. The surgeon was confident, however, that there was no danger of metastatic disease, even though I had had cancer before. He advised and I chose to take no chemotherapy.

Recovery was slow. I was afraid to turn over or sit up or walk because I could feel everything shift inside me. When I started eating again, it involved great pain, and nausea became a regular part of my day. So did diarrhea and the weakness that came with it. I had no clothes that fit. I remember trying on a blouse in a clothing store one day and turning around to see a large lump on my left back. I panicked and thought I had another tumor. When I reached for it, I was embarrassed to find it was my shoulder blade! My body had become a stranger to me.

I went back to work before I had planned and proceeded to live my life. In the meantime, I learned that my mother had taken DES when she was pregnant with me. I also learned that girls and women whose mothers took DES developed cervical and ovarian cancer more often than those who did not. I have learned that this is now also true for grandchildren of women who took DES. It was at this time that I decided that I would not choose to have children. It was far too risky.

Still, I felt I had been lucky. I was alive, reasonably healthy, and often pain free. I really thought I had had my last round with cancer and that I had won. It was great!

One year and three months later (January 1980), I noticed I felt a definite lack of energy. I felt sick and weak and had this swollen gland in my armpit. It would not go away. By this time I had found a wonderful doctor who listened to me and believed what I had to say. I went to see him. He did a biopsy and blood tests. He immediately sent me to an oncologist who was to diagnose this as a form of non-Hodgkin's lymphoma. He told me that there were many people who survive this disease on their own, but there were few truly effective treatments. He also suggested that I might become a part of an experimental program that was testing Interferon, a relatively new drug that had lower toxicity and was to be the wonder drug of the 1980s. It was hoped that this drug would cure everything from cancer to the common cold.

I cannot now describe the fear I felt then. I felt totally and completely alone and I was terrified! The doctor put me in touch with the local chapter of the American Cancer Society. I have very little good to say about ACS, but this local group was doing wonderful things. They provided me with an "advocate" who would be available at the drop of a hat to take me here or there, give advice, listen.[*] I did not use this resource as much as I might have, but I did get some very helpful information from her. She told me about a group that met once each week—a cancer survivors' group. Everyone in the group was in treat-

---

[*] This is one of the services some of the grassroots women's cancer projects are now trying to implement.

ment for cancer; I could go, observe, participate while I decided what I wanted to do.

This group of people, and the things I learned from them, saved my life. I truly believe this. I agreed to treatment with Interferon, I went to this group, and I started to believe that I would survive.

Chemotherapy was hard. I did not lose much hair. Nor did I have to spend time in the hospital. I did lose weight, and was sick much of the time. And my physical strength waned badly. I also had pneumonia several times that winter. But I did believe that I would win. I did not think I would die, or that I wanted to die, but rather chose to live. I learned breathing techniques that would help with the pain and nausea. I learned to visualize myself as a healthy, whole person. I learned to meditate for the calm it could bring me. And I went into remission, got sick again, back and forth, back and forth. My last chemotherapy treatment was in May 1983. I felt this remission was permanent.

The remission has lasted and I continue to feel that it will last. I learned a lot about myself and the importance of mind over body. I do not believe that people choose to be ill. I do believe that people who are ill can choose to die and that dying is not necessarily losing. I also believe that people can learn a lot from illness. I feel I have and I continue to be challenged by my experiences.

This story is not quite finished. During the summer of 1985, my doctor found a spot under my arm. It was a small patch of discolored, rough skin. When removed and biopsied, it was found to be a simple skin cancer—of little concern except for my history and the fact that it was in my armpit. My doctor suggested some radiation to make sure it was gone. That last treatment was August 16, 1985. I have met and passed the five-year mark that seems so important. I have survived.

I have learned something about cancer. Not about biology, but about people and cancer. I will forever see cancer as an issue for women, because the people I knew best who had cancer were women. Each year there are more women diagnosed with breast cancer than there are people who have died of AIDS since our first knowledge of this disease in the United States. Also, people with cancer are often invisible. Friends don't want to hear about cancer because they are afraid.

I have learned about women who were forced to quit their jobs because they had cancer. Without jobs, there is no insurance, and without insurance, there is often less intensive treatment. And support services are not there if you cannot afford to pay for them. Because women are often at the bottom of the economic ladder, they are the least able to pay, and often with children, the most in need.

I have learned about strength, especially my own. I know that it takes real strength to admit the need for help. It takes real strength to help a friend in terrible pain die on her own terms. It takes real strength to grow through pain and outlast it. And it takes strength to recover, because recovery is slow and arduous, and often more work than giving in and letting go.

Again this summer and this fall and this winter I have had scares. Problems with my body that have been checked for cancer: a small lump in my heel, swollen glands, nearly continuous uterine bleeding. In each case these were considered more dangerous because of my cancer history. And in each case there has been a verdict of "not cancer" and a sigh of relief, along with yet another celebration. I have gotten on with my life. But in my life there will always be the specter of what might have been along with the corresponding fear of what may yet be. And I continue to tell myself that this is truly no big deal.

Thoughts on Cancer & Healing

Selma Miriam

Experience with cancer is a shock. It makes one consider, as never before, what dying will be like (and therefore what one's living has been), as well as confronting one with the ludicrousness of our medical care.

My own experience was in 1978, and I seem to have survived. A year previous I had started, with other women, a feminist restaurant and bookstore. At the beginning, this dream of ours required my skills, and I had invested in it all my money. There was no way I could do what the doctors required— that is, to get a mastectomy—because I couldn't afford that time in the hospital without the death of the dream. With Audre Lorde's phrase "We were not meant to survive" ringing in my mind, I refused the mastectomy (after an "excision biopsy" of a small lump in my breast was found to be malignant), but I did agree to go for radiation. It was five days a week for six weeks. The doctors had said there would be no side effects beyond unusual tiredness. When I experienced worse than that, they didn't want to hear about it. They lied to me, were sometimes kind and sometimes sadistic. As I sat in the endless waiting rooms, sometimes with very small children with tumors, I couldn't help but resent the comments from the new age types who frequented our vegetarian restaurant that it was stress that caused cancer. What about these kids? And as for my rage, I treasured it!

Because we were doing so many things differently, we developed procedures during this time that I think were very useful and should be considered by any woman who is sick. Most importantly, I never went to a doctor alone, including into the examining room. We even demanded, when my lymph nodes were to be surgically examined, that I be under local anesthesia and that two of my friends be in the operating room. A different friend went with me each of the five days a week for the six weeks for the radiation. It's an amazing reality check, both for the doctor and for the patient! We now do it whenever any of us needs medical care. And we won't go to any doctor who doesn't accept it.

Because of the onslaught of opinions on how to deal with cancer, it was necessary to weed through my "friends." This my partners helped me to do. While I didn't mind chewing apricot pits (which supposedly contained Laetrile—popular in the seventies) or eating sprouted seeds each morning, there were some whose opinions or advice were intolerable, and when they got too insistent in our public space (the restaurant), they had to be told to leave. It was too hard, physically and emotionally, to have to listen to them. My partners were invaluable at this time.

In 1980 my mother died in a hospital. She didn't die of cancer and she was 82 years old. But in the six weeks of her hospital stay, I watched in horror at just how bad the doctors were—their lies, their mistakes, and the resulting unnecessary pain she went through. After this, I dropped my health insurance. During my cancer experience, I'd had to decide that I was going to die one day anyway and that I couldn't let them hold that fact over my head while they insisted on doing (or experimenting) as they saw fit. Insurance money lets them do this. Since I had decided never to go back to Yale Medical after their lies, I didn't need the insurance.

Since then, we've found there are other kinds of healing, and insurance usually doesn't pay for it anyway. Homeopathy took care of a funny cramping pain in my ovary and at the same time all those "benign" lumps in my breasts and in my underarm lymph nodes disappeared. These days we go to homeopathic doctors or acupuncturists. These are older, kinder, and effective methods of healing!

In 1984 I tried to think about grief. I had lost a lover that year, and my father had died and all these experiences needed to be considered in a different light. I wrote the following pieces, which we published in our cookbook *The Second Seasonal Political Palate.**

A Witch Recipe for Grievers

Sometimes nothing can be done to change things, and hurt and anger must be transmuted: Examples include the death of someone loved, permanent body damage like breast cancer, dissolution of relationships. See what you can use from this "recipe."

1. In the middle of the worst pain, try to find something to make, to create for yourself something difficult and particularly rewarding. Even if you can't start it now, plan to start it soon. Something that will last. Write something, sew something. Use your own special, already polished skill to plan and create a lasting present for yourself. Women used to make mourning quilts and embroideries. (See Judy Chicago's *Embroidering Our Heritage.*)

---

* *The Second Seasonal Political Palate,* by the Bloodroot Collective, Bridgeport, CT: Sanguinaria Publishers, 1984.

2. Consider your friends. Withdraw from the ones who are frightened by your pain, the ones who think there might have been something you could have done, should still do to change things, the ones who want to be "fair." Remember you have a right to judge and to be angry. Don't forget Hecate. When you're hurting, you need especially considerate tenderness. As lonely as you may feel, it's better to have fewer or no friends than those who won't care to understand. Perhaps it is fear of friends' lack of sensitivity which sends so many women to therapists—to pay for a supposedly nonjudgmental caring with a hidden agenda of "fitting" into the therapist's norms, whatever those may be.

3. Take charge of your sorrow. It will take some time to project ahead and think when the pain will be over, but with effort, you'll be able to see that end. Pain comes in and out like waves. When it recedes, you may feel it is over. Then another wave engulfs you: that's when you must remember that there will be a time when it will be past— a time you can name. Not next week, not next month. Maybe in three months. Maybe not until fall or spring. Whenever it is, set it as a goal. Know you can survive until then. Meanwhile, take the time between to make an ending ritual. Jews burn a candle for eight days after a loved one dies. The candle is in a tall glass, and as the flame burns lower the upper part of the glass darkens until the flame goes out by itself and the glass is all dark. Other candles are lit on the anniversary of the death and on particular holidays.

Create a ritual. Remember—a ritual has symbolic meaning—so whatever you chose to do must have significance for you. And a ritual must be repetitive. You must be able to do it again and again—time when you don't seem to need it, and times when you can't imagine that it will help. For example—a candle can be marked off in days and burned, a little each day. Maybe pictures or letters should be burned, or if you prefer, torn in small pieces and sent off in running water—a little each day or week until the bad time is past. Sometimes anger requires a hex. Remember, Z Budapest has said a witch that cannot hex cannot heal.

4. Remember the healing power of work, if it is work you love and in which you believe. Remember a feminist is a woman who recognizes the common oppression of women and will struggle against it. We need to imagine repairing, reweaving, mending the damage done, as Mary Daly points out, and then to do it.

How To Be a Griever's Friend

A griever's friend is one who is there, who spends more time than seems reasonable with a griever. She listens and understands. She isn't Polyanna. She's angry at her friend's pain. She values loyalty over fairness. She doesn't say "You should have" or "Why didn't you" or "How you should," and she tries not to let the griever think that way about herself. She tells the griever over and over that what has happened is not fair, not deserved; that anger is justified.

A Note on Dying

Maybe it is not until our own death becomes imminent, palpable, that we can consider how we live. Those of us who have been told we have some fatal disease are faced with choices about our living, now. Of course, we all know someday we will die, yet we don't know it until living is thrown into sharp focus, whether it is daily behavior or what we let the doctors do to delay the event. Certainly the one in four women with breast cancer must face this reality. Those of us who have spent time with someone dying, when it is not taken entirely from our hands by the medical profession, and when it is not sudden and/or violent, know that it is a transformation that possesses its own wonder, triumph, and joy.

REFERENCES

Lorde, Audre, *The Cancer Journals*, 2nd edition (San Francisco, CA: Spinster Aunt Lute, 1980).

Lorde, Audre, "A Litany for Survival" in *The Black Unicorn* (New York: Norton, 1978).

Gray, Elizabeth Dodson, *Green Paradise Lost* (Wellesley, MA: Roundtable Press, 1979).

Starhawk, *Dreaming the Dark* (Boston: Beacon Press, 1989).

From a Cancer Journal

Merida Wexler

I have cancer. The ground opens beneath my feet. A single swift abduction—even as narcissus and purple hyacinth bloom in my spring garden. I feel maiden—taken irrevocably. I tumble into the icy grip of death.

▲ ▲ ▲

I lie in the warm soapy bath water caressing my belly. I talk to the cancer in my cervix. Who are you? How long have you been here? Why? Why? Why? She doesn't answer questions. I sink more deeply into watery warmth; begin to listen through my hands. I can feel her ache now. And then I see her. She is a flower! A rose. Black-red petals thick and dry as scabs. But a bloom, yes, she is a bloom. Life, not death, but life growing here. I lay warm hands gently around her. Softly I say "I'm here now."

▲ ▲ ▲

This is life that could become death. This bloom here at life's gateway. To carry death where I've carried life—yes, that I understand. Deathlife gathered together at the same gate. Have I planted her as once I planted my babies? Does she grow from my wishes? My wounds? Has the weight of my terrors fed her? Oh gateway to life and death, you are not numbly neutral, do not mechanically open and shut. She opens from the heart, from the clit. From desire. She opens ferociously, wide beyond imagining, to life. And now she has opened to this cancer flower. She carries this too. Another and another of what

53

dwells here. But I will not give birth to my death. Not yet. Not here.

▲ ▲ ▲

At 3 AM I wake in a pool of blood. Is it my period or has the tumor ruptured? Oh, terror! But this blood between my legs—how can I be afraid of it? So many years, so familiar. Joe wakes, wraps warm arms around me (so many years). His soft voice in my ear. And new fear flooding his loving eyes. Hold me! The other night I lay in a circle of my dear woman friends. Their hands, hands that washed Vivian's dead body, stay steady on me as I squirm and scream, choke on my horror. Later in the dark of the sweatlodge, I sit slippery with fear, close by these loved and loving women, familiar as sweat, singing prayers. Hold me close!

▲ ▲ ▲

I'm learning that I am a touchstone for others' terror. Cancer afflicts all of us. The fear of contagion; the grief of losses known. I'm charged with the evocative power of this disease. Strangers throw advice at me as if spraying me with disinfectant. Read this. Eat this. This will cure. This cause. So certain? It's different inside the disease. I'm asked, "Why you? Why cervical cancer? What does it mean?" I say: cancer means cancer. It means itself. I learn 'meaning' takes me away from the cancer; distances me from the truth of what occurs. Simone Weil has written: "Prayer consists of attention." Yes. This is what I try to do. I attend. I stay with myself. This is the gift of cancer: to be present with myself, to not abandon myself, no matter what. To be present with the 3 AM terrors, present for the loving touch, present under the daily radiation. I stay with her, with me.

▲ ▲ ▲

Staying present leads me to new ways of meditating. I can't send aggression into my body. Especially not here—my womb, my cervix, my vagina. They've known too much hate and violence. However, I do have my totem animal. The polar bear I saw at the zoo three days after I found out. There we were, both in our cages. The bear looked at me with such calmness, looking out from within himself. The equanimity of his gaze held me. That and his immense beauty—such white, white fur and so black his eyes, nose, paw pads. Sometimes on my walk home after radiation I see him. And I feed him lots of cancer fish! He doesn't have to hunt; to slash and kill. It's a free meal! Sometimes he curls up in me and sleeps.

▲ ▲ ▲

I don't recognize this blood I squeeze from the sponge. Gone the black-red menses, the thick clots. This is thin, brownish, mixed with the blood from the tumor. Death blood, life blood. Both exhausted. This last blood expiring from my womb.

▲ ▲ ▲

Friday evening after work. Walgreen's. A pick-up truck parks in front of me. I read the bumper sticker: Shit Happens. I laugh, enjoying the matter-of-fact tone. Buddhism's First Noble Truth in slang. I think of the nurse who draws my blood. She's deeply tanned in February. How ironic her choosing an irradiated sun-bed tan and weekly monitoring radiation-sickened blood. I dismiss her as a pleasant air-head with no troubles. Ah, the aggrandizement of cancer! She misses one week and on her return I ask if she were sick. "No," she says, "My daughter had two grand mal seizures that day." I learn she's given one of her kidneys to this ailing child. Oh, the commonplace of suffering. A good cleansing pie in the face for my pretentiousness! Shit happens.

▲ ▲ ▲

I will have to have a hysterectomy. I will lose my beloved. On the summer solstice. A ceremony of sacrifice. My womb offered to the sun. One vessel of life taken so the greater vessel of life may continue. This is such grief! Sacrifice, I remember, means to make sacred. What am I sacred-making? All I feel is the huge loss. I cannot keep life by holding. I can only keep life by giving life away. And I can't even know what will be beyond this giving. Life? Death? Can I give this? Is it sacred-making when it is taken not given?

▲ ▲ ▲

Tomorrow they will take you out. Can you still hear me, sweetie? I croon to you . . . Tell me all you know, I will remember it always. Oh, toots, I rub your golden belly lamp. You who have been with me from the beginning. Womb heart of my deepest place. I slip my fingers inside and tickle her. We laugh together. Oh beauty, oh sweetie, you are more than cells to me. I will have a phantom womb. I will re-member you—as amputees stand on the lost leg.

▲ ▲ ▲

When I tell the doctor I want my womb, he tells me I can't have it. Something about documenting the cancer. Oh, come on! All those hysterectomies. There must be one helluva building to hold all the wombs. Well, I will go visit her at the lab and say goodbye. At the front desk the receptionist drops her smile, tells me to have a seat. Disappears. Returns to usher me into the lab. I'm quite a sensation. Am I the first woman to come to see her womb? Heads turn; white coats hover nearby. One brings me my womb. In a zip-lock bag! Oh my, she looks like sushi—so many cross-sections sliced out for slides. Everyone's watching me. I can't say goodbye to her here. So I begin to talk with the tech. "You really keep this forever?" "Oh no, we keep the slides. We'll throw this out in two months." "I want it." Now I've really created a sensation! They all look at each other, but no one can think of a reason to refuse. The tech writes SAVE on the label. As I turn to leave she asks, "Excuse me, but why do you want it?" . . . She was part of me, she held my children, she sang when I came, I loved her. . . . Aloud I mutter some small words. But when our eyes meet I think: she knows why.

▲ ▲ ▲

Shadows. So many shadows here on the other side of cancer. This borderland I cross is full of fears. Did they get it all? Will it come back? Will it kill me? What if . . .? No! I did not have cancer to be afraid of getting cancer. If it comes back, I'll take care of it then. But I will not spend all my days peering into shadows. Scram!

▲ ▲ ▲

My friend asks me what I need to continue my healing. Now almost a year after cancer. Without reflection, instinctively, I say "Desire." I don't mean desire to heal—of course that. But desire. I want desire. Desire heals. When she lives in me I'm healed. I sicken when she is gone. She flickers in me these days, a warm wan light. Coming closer. At last! Perhaps she is my phantom womb. Yes! This is the sacred-making. How she heals me.

Fighting Spirit

Nancy Lanoue[*]

Osu! Kaicho, Senseis, and Senpais.[**] I am very grateful for the opportunity to be with you all today. The three years since I last stood in this position have brought many unexpected changes to my life which have both affected and been affected by my practice of karate. In my nidan promotion essay, I wrote about the experience of starting a school and learning how to train alone. The spirit I felt then was one of pride and satisfaction at having accomplished something that had been difficult for me. Little did I know that far greater challenges lay ahead.

In May of 1987, a week before my thirty-fifth birthday, I was diagnosed with breast cancer. I remember distinctly receiving a call from my doctor with this news, and then five minutes later going upstairs to teach a class. What a wonderful blessing it was to have karate in my life at that moment. As we sat seiza[***] and the student volunteer called

---

[*] Nancy Lanoue and her life partner Jeannette Pappas opened the Women's Gym in Chicago in 1985; they closed it 1989 when Jeannette's need for cancer treatment necessitated it. Nancy is currently teaching karate and self-defense to women and children, as director of Chicago Women's Seido Karate Center. She wrote this essay in March 1990 as part of her promotion examination for 3rd degree black belt.

[**] *Osu* is a Japanese word that means "to continue to strive—with patience." It is used as a respectful greeting among martial artists. *Kaicho* means grandmaster; *sensei* means teacher; and *senpai* means senior.

[***] *Seiza* refers to the traditional, formal Japanese way of sitting on folded legs.

mokuso,* I wondered if everyone could hear my heart pounding and see the fear of death in my eyes. When we rose to begin, panic started to consume me, but then a fighting spirit sharpened by ten years of training took me over and made me shout YOI!** Our familiar ritual of getting ready took on new meaning for me at that moment, and as I started to punch, kick, and kiai*** with my students, I let myself hope and then finally believe that I would be able to fight my cancer.

Three weeks later I entered the hospital to have a mastectomy. As I was waking from the effects of the anesthesia, I felt a strong pressure in my chest and looked down to see a tightly wrapped bandage encircling my body from my armpits to almost my waist. This didn't alarm me because I had prepared myself for a taut flatness where my breast had been. What did frighten me was that I couldn't lift my left arm any higher than my shoulder. As it turned out, the main vein to my arm was accidently severed when the surgeon made his first incision and had to be sewn back together again. This would make my recovery slower and more difficult, I was told, but I could still expect to regain more or less "full use of my arm."

As I lay there unable to breathe deeply or move without pain, it occurred to me that my understanding of the phrase "full use" might be very different from the doctor's. To me, full use meant being able

---

* *Mokuso* means "begin meditation."

** *Yoi* means "get ready." At that command, everyone breathes deeply in and then forcefully out while tightening the muscles in the core of the body. The purpose is to help one become grounded, with concentration, fully present in the moment.

*** *Kiai* means "yell of spirit." It serves to frighten the opponent and activate the fighting spirit.

to do one arm pushups and to punch with enough speed and focus to hear my gi[*] snap. To me, full range of motion meant being able to do the big, round Seido version of the shuto mawashi uke[**] which I had always told my students they must do perfectly because it is the most aesthetically beautiful move in our movement vocabulary.

Every medical person I tried to speak to about my concerns looked baffled and slightly shocked, especially the sweet Reach-for-Recovery volunteer who told me proudly that after doing her rehab exercises faithfully, she could now comb her hair without pain and reach things on even the highest shelf in her kitchen.

The next day I resolved to begin working on regaining my strength and range of motion in my arm. At first, I tried the various climb-the-wall-with-your-fingers exercises I had been shown. But after an hour of little success and much pain, I snuck down the hall to an empty corridor carrying my I.V. pole and surgery drainage bag with me to try another approach.

There I secretly began practicing Yansu,[***] at first with great hesitation and doubt, but then increasingly with joy and a deep gratitude that I was alive and could move at all. I have always loved this particular kata[+] and felt that it nurtures a deep sense of balance and wholeness within the body. For me that day it served that purpose, with my strong right

---

[*] *Gi* means karate uniform.

[**] *Shuto mawashi uke* means roundhouse knifehand block.

[***] *Yansu* is a form all Seido karate students learn at green belt. Its name means "keep pure."

[+] *Kata* literally means "form." Katas are choreographed exercises practiced by most martial artists in which the movements tell the story of an imaginary battle with multiple opponents.

side lending energy to my struggling left so that
both could work together to create the beautiful
push/pull beginning of double ridgehand, double
punch, right and left inverted strike, right and left
vertical spearhand, KIAI! I still don't fully understand how or why, but doing Yansu in my hospital
gown with tubes and poles in the way everywhere
started a physical and emotional healing process in
me that I will always be grateful for.

For a few months after surgery, it continued to be
painful to move my arm into full extension or to do
movements with full power. I can't say that I wel-
comed it, but the experience of training with chronic
pain did have its benefits. It was the first time I had
ever experienced such a powerful physical limita-
tion, the first time I simply could not make my body
do what I wanted it to do. I think it has made me a
better teacher because I now realize what it actually
feels like to be physically challenged. It is not fun to
train when you are in pain, and students with special challenges need a lot of support and
encouragement as they push into and finally
through their pain.

At the recommendation of my doctors, I underwent an aggressive course of chemotherapy during
the late summer and fall of 1987. The theory behind
it is that the chemotherapy will kill off any remaining cancer cells that may still be in the body after
surgery. In practice, it makes one quite sick, and in
my case, made all my hair fall out leaving me
utterly bald without even eyebrows, eyelashes, or
body hair. I stayed this way for approximately six
months until the treatments were over and my hair
began to grow back in.

During my whole cancer experience, I thought
many times of Kaicho's lesson that it is not the obstacles or challenges we have that are meaningful, but

rather our responses to them. For me, the challenge of cancer created an opportunity for growth by presenting issues on which I had to take a stand, knowing full well that my choices were both personal and political.

One out of ten women will get breast cancer some time in her life, and yet we never know who each other are because we are invisible to one another. It is assumed that we will wear a prosthesis (a false breast) or that we will undergo another major surgery to have our breast "reconstructed." In fact, women with breast cancer are inundated with information about what are really only cosmetic solutions to this life-threatening problem. My Reach-for-Recovery volunteer reassured me that with a prosthesis, "no one will ever know what happened." My response to this was firstly, why would I want to pretend that it had never happened; secondly, what right does anyone have to ask me to do that; and finally, how would any of the lessons that may come of this get passed on to other people happen if I did that?

I agree with the black lesbian poet, Audre Lorde, herself a cancer survivor, who has said: "Well,women with breast cancer are warriors, also. I have been to war, and still am. So has every woman who has one or both breasts amputated because of the cancer that is becoming the primary physical scourge of our time. For me, my scars are an honorable reminder that I may be a casualty in the cosmic war against radiation, animal fat, air pollution, McDonald's hamburgers, and Red Dye No. 2, but the fight is still going on, and I am still a part of it ... I refuse to be reduced in my own eyes or in the eyes of others from warrior to mere victim, simply because it might render me a fraction more acceptable or less dangerous to the still complacent, those who believe that if you cover up a problem it ceases to exist."[*]

This same issue came up again when the choice presented itself to wear a wig or not to wear a wig. I chose not to, partly because I was sure it would fall off when I was teaching or training, but also because, like Audre Lorde, I didn't want to become invisible.

Instead I became an oddball for the first time in my life. And I learned what it feels like to be different, unable to fit in. People's reaction to my baldness ran the gamut from mild curiosity to strong disapproval. A surprising number assumed I had done it for fashion and reproached me for being so wild. In retrospect, I can see that even these painful encounters provided opportunities for learning and sharing.

For me, losing my hair meant having nothing left to physically hide behind, and it has helped me let go of the emotional armor I used to hide behind as well. It has made me more open, more willing to just put out there who I am and what I have to offer, and assume people will either take it or leave it. By making me a little less afraid of disapproval, being involuntarily bald has been liberating.

Last spring, almost two years after my diagnosis, my life partner Jeannette Pappas was found to have inoperable pancreatic cancer. She was 46 years old. Unlike my situation which had a fairly hopeful prognosis, extensive research failed to turn up even one long-term survivor of Jeannette's type of cancer through traditional cancer therapies.

Together we made the difficult decision to close the Women's Gym which we had struggled for three years to create and four years to keep running, in

---

[*] Audre Lorde, *The Cancer Journals* (San Francisco: Spinsters/Aunt Lute Book Company, 1980), p. 60.

order to go to California to pursue an experimental radiation therapy which was offered there. It was painful to leave my students, especially the seniors who at this point were second kyu[*] brown belts, without any sense of when, if ever, I would have the opportunity to teach again. But I would never have had such a beautiful school in the first place if it hadn't been for Jeannette's immeasurable talent, energy, and devotion. My decision to be 100-percent with her through this ordeal flowed naturally from the situation. Throughout the summer, Jeannette was a model of what Kaicho has called non-quitting spirit. Several times each day we practiced zazen[**] together for the dual purpose of controlling our fear and in her case, becoming strong enough to live with intense pain. Up until one month before she died, she refused all pain medicine, despite her doctor's pleas, saying that it prevented her from being fully present and awake to what was happening each moment.

I had found two teacups with the image of Daruma[***] on them, and each morning we silently drank in the familiar message: seven times fall down, eight times get up. Then we would go outside the cabin where we were staying, and I would help push or pull Jeannette, who was quite weak at this point, up the steep hill to our car for the daily drive to Berkeley. She was the only patient at this center who never missed one treatment. Once she had chosen her path, she stuck to it with an iron

---

[*] Second kyu is a rank two levels below black belt.

[**] *Zazen* refers to sitting meditation practice.

[***] *Daruma* is the Japanese name for Bodhidarm, the legendary Indian monk who founded Buddhism and brought it to China in the sixth century A.D. The Shaolin monastery he established there was a center for the development and practice of martial arts for many centuries.

will, announcing at the end of her life that she had
no regrets about her treatment even though it
seemed not to have helped her because she had
approached it with all the hope in the world and
had given 100-percent effort. As Jeannette's time
grew shorter, she came more and more to exemplify
what I see as the path to true warriorship. The late
Tibetan Buddhist teacher Chogyam Trungpa
Rinpoche has said: "To be a warrior is to learn to be
genuine in every moment of your life."[*] Jeannette's
way of doing this was to consciously shed the
facade of tough emotional armor that had protected
her through 46 years of hard living. She contacted
all the people from her past with whom she had
unresolved issues and tried to heal old wounds.
Instead of closing off and pulling into herself as so
many dying people seem to do, she opened up and
fervently tried to extend her belief that death was a
transition rather than an ending to those of us who
needed to hear this in order to let her go. She also
took care of all the business related to her funeral
and property disposition so that the burden would
not fall on those she loved. When I would marvel at
the way she had chosen finally to live and die, she
told me it was her way of expressing fighting spirit.
I have tried to learn from her and to incorporate this
deeper understanding of spirit in my own training
and teaching.

It is five months exactly since Jeannette's death. I
have returned to teaching full time and have even
made plans to start a children's karate program next

---

[*] Chogyam Trungpa, *Shambhala: The Sacred Path of the Warrior*
(Boston: Shambhala Publications, 1984), p. 70.

month. My senior students are now first kyus,* and I am anxiously but happily preparing them to test for shodan in the fall.** Just last week I was honored to be selected to teach at the Special Training camp sponsored by the National Martial Arts Federation to be held in New Haven, Connecticut this coming July. On one level, I seem to have survived this last crisis and to be functioning fairly productively. But on another level, I feel weak and vulnerable and more wounded than I can ever explain.

Every single day it is a struggle to find the will to move toward life and to believe that doom is not just around the corner. I have been in the caretaker mode for so long that I have trouble remembering that it's me who needs loving care now. When Kaicho asked me to try to prepare for this promotion, I was shocked because I have done so little physical training this past year. Now I believe that is exactly why I was given this particular challenge now: as an incentive and opportunity to put my focus back on myself where it must be if I am to heal and become whole again.

To make up for not being able to train at Honbu,*** I often inspire myself by watching the video of the 1986 Black Belt demonstration. So many sounds and images from it bring up loving memories for me: Sensei Ken's wise and witty commentary; Senseis Newton and Sana making even the most impossible moves look effortless; my first Seido training bud-

---

* First kyu is one level below black belt.

** My four senior students did finally attain black belt on September 23, 1990.

*** *Honbu* means "headquarters." It refers to my teacher's school in New York City.

dies Senpais Sue Koch and Debra Hershkowitz proving that women's kumite* can be every bit as interesting and dynamic as men's; Senpai Judy sending the biggest men imaginable rolling and tumbling like bowling pins; Sensei Solly's dignity; Kaicho with his tonfa** moving like a graceful, lethal jungle cat.

All of these images and many more live in my heart and mind and have helped sustain my connection to karate through these difficult times. But the one image that has held the deepest meaning for me personally is that of Sensei Jean Battle doing Seienchin kata.*** My understanding of this form is that is speaks of endurance and survival: the capacity to sustain strength and spirit over a long period of time. This is my only training goal right now. Every time I see Sensei Jean or watch her do this kata, I get closer to believing that it is possible.

---

*   *Kumite* is unchoreographed sparring or free-fighting.

**   The *tonfa* is a traditional martial arts weapon.

*** Sensei Jean Battle is the most senior woman in the Seido Karate organization. Her husband, Charles Battle, was a beloved Seido teacher who died suddenly, at a very young age, on Christmas Eve in 1980, leaving Sensei Jean with two young children to raise alone.

My Body: A Map of Memories

Ada Harrigan

After living in New York for nine years, on and off, I was stumped as to whether there was both a West Broadway and a Broadway. I hadn't checked a map before leaving home so I approached a stranger who confirmed that both existed and he sent me off in the right direction. It was my first appointment and I didn't want to be even a few minutes late.

I entered the office reception area and was given a clipboard and a questionnaire to complete. When and how did my grandparents die? The grandmother I never met died of breast cancer at 36. She was on my father's side, so I'd been told not to worry. What was my own health history? The usual questions.

"Ahdah Harringan" called out an assistant, mispronouncing my name. I followed her to an examining room. She pointed to a rose colored robe on the table and said "everything off and put that on."

After she shut the door, I panicked and followed her into the hallway asking "which side goes in front?" With that answered, I returned to the room and disrobed. I sat on a chair in the corner. My feet were cold on the bare linoleum.

What am I doing here alone? Don't you ever learn? Voices in my head reprimanded me. I had made a pledge to myself during my earlier illnesses that I would always take my partner or a friend with me to doctor's appointments. I've received enough bad news to appreciate the immediate presence of a handholder.

I was glancing through *People* magazine when Dr. Borden entered. She was popular with a number of women I knew who referred to her by her first name, Robin, even though their only contact with her was as a health professional. A small, trim, attractive woman, she had an efficient, professional demeanor.

After a brief hello she glanced at my chart and repeated the facts. "Hodgkin's disease twice, chemotherapy in '87, no periods since last April, hot flashes for the past four months."

"There's something else," I replied while shaking inside, hoping to stifle the tears in my eyes. "I started recovering incest memories last April and I never had a period again. My period did stop during chemotherapy but it started again. I'd had it for a year prior to the memories." Robin shook her head with dismay. "I feel there's a relationship between the incest and my cancer." She heard what I said but didn't respond.

Before I got on the table I requested the smallest speculum. I usually forget to ask and they start out with one that's too big and pinches me. I don't know if my size has to do with lack of intercourse, lack of childbearing, or is just bone structure. I think of myself as big boned because of my broad shoulders but my hands are small and when I got braces my orthodontist had to pull four molars in order to get the others straight. He said I had too many teeth for my jaw.

I approached the table barefoot, and Robin suggested I would be more comfortable with my shoes on. I followed instructions and stepped into the stirrups.

"If you want me to stop at any time, just tell me and I will."

On hearing her say this I felt relieved at my options. I'm not sure when we picked up the conversation.

"Are there other children?" she asked.

"Yes. I have an older sister. I know he got her too. She's in some of my memories. She's labeled schizophrenic and is in a mental hospital right now. She's been in and out several times. My brother was abused too. So far his memories have to do with older boys in the neighborhood. He's diagnosed as depressed and was in the hospital for a while too. Now he's on medication and living with my parents. He's 36. He called me and told me he believes me and related how one time when my sister was having one of her so-called 'spells' she yelled out 'keep dad away from me; he wants to have sex with me!' My mother tries to calm her down when she lives with them. Tells her it's just her imagination. It's not. It's her memories of terror and rape. My brother is living with them now. He said he doesn't know what to do. He's not working and he's dependent on my parents."

"So you've confronted the abuser?"

"Yes. My dad. The first week I remembered I phoned and confronted him. He denied it. I have a younger sister too. She's getting married in a few weeks. I didn't even get an invitation. They say I'm crazy. That it is not true. That I've been through so much I've snapped." I started crying. I felt totally abandoned and alone, unloved and denied.

Dr. Borden looked directly at me and said, "you still need validation."

I felt like a little girl. I didn't ask her what she meant. I had read about stages of recovery. Stage one for me was the emergency stage as described by Ellen Bass and Laura Davis in *The Courage To Heal*. Fortunately that stage was over, but what was next?

The prior Friday night I had gone to a survivors' group for women. I had called the incest survivor's hotline and the recorded message said the meeting began at seven but when I arrived it was well under-way and I later learned that a few weeks earlier the group had changed the starting time to 6:30. I men-tioned to Robin how much it had disturbed me to attend this meeting. It was called twelve-step, but my experience was as a no-step. There was a time-keeper who signalled to each speaker when her time was up. My worst nightmares come true were shared one after the other until 7:55 when we said the serenity prayer and disbursed. There was no lit-erature, no apparent host, and it was one of those anonymous meetings. Was speaking to others out-side that room against the rules? What were the rules?

After the meeting I fell into a deep depression that lasted for weeks. I didn't return. I had attended the meeting anticipating that I would feel better and instead I felt worse.

Later, in Dr. Borden's office, she told me I should go again and arrive early. She had heard it was a good group from a number of women.

During the examination, Borden told me that I didn't look menopausal since I was lubricated. One effect of menopause is vaginal dryness.

"Are you seeing anyone?" she asked.

"Yes. I have a lover."

"When did you last have sex?"

"I don't remember. It's been months. I guess it's psychological. When I start getting affectionate I just want to hit, slug somebody. But mostly I feel like my emotions are submerged. I feel anger, rage, and dev-astation, but that's about it."

Dr. Borden told me the only way to be certain as to whether or not I was menopausal was to have a blood test. I left my body momentarily at the mention of it. Eight months of chemotherapy with each treatment preceded by blood tests had collapsed and scarred my veins. My treatments were injected through the wrist area and the back of my hands. I had felt my veins burning from the drugs. The lack of good veins extends from my fingers to my upper arms.

One memory flashed through my body. I was in Portland at my oncologist's and I had said "no blood tests" but I had been talked into it. The lab was adjacent to his waiting room and they always left the door open while they worked. The assistant jabbed me several times with the needle, apologizing profusely for the pain she was inflicting. Once she must have hit a nerve. A primal scream came out of my mouth and I felt my body rise from the chair. The scream was audible to the entire waiting room. My lover, who had been waiting outside, ran in and put her arm on my shoulders. I was crying from the jolt and I was angry that my arms had been destroyed in the course of my cancer treatments. I remember the smell of that place. I hated it.

Robin told me she'd meet me in her office. Shortly, an assistant arrived to draw blood. I braced myself and took a deep breath. "I don't have any good veins," I told her. "The last time they attempted to draw blood they tried five different places and didn't get any." She pressed on the inside on my elbow and looked perplexed.

"I'd better get someone with more experience," she said and left the room.

She returned with an older woman who proceeded in the same manner. The new arrival put a tourniquet on my arm and had me make a fist and release several times. She kept shaking her head back and forth.

"Un uh," she said, shaking her head back and forth indicating a lack of a target for the needle.

There was one area that she thought might be productive but she didn't want to attempt it. "Dr. Borden's going to have to do this one," she sighed.

The way she looked at me made me very uncomfortable. What's she think I'm a junkie or something? So my arms aren't normal. Give me a break.

I was led into the hall and directed to sit on a high chair facing a counter. A few minutes later Borden appeared and it was déjà vu. Tourniquet on the arm, make fist and release, veins get prodded, deep sighs from the medical professional. She decided on a spot below my thumb. I couldn't see a vein and I hoped she was right. She used a butterfly, a tiny, flexible tube attached to a vial. I looked away. I felt a sting. I won't cry, I told myself. It seemed like minutes passed. I looked down and I could see there was some blood in the tiny tube but none in the vial. Was Borden frustrated? I closed my eyes and visualized a full tube of blood.

"Thank you," said Dr. Borden.

I looked down and saw the vial filling up. "I was visualizing," I replied.

"Well it worked."

"Gosh, no one's been able to get blood out of me for a while. I think you should test everything now that we've got some." I filled two vials with blood and Robin instructed the assistants on the tests to be ordered.

With that ordeal complete, I followed Robin to her office. She explained estrogen replacement therapy and why she was a proponent. A younger friend of mine had recommended it and also told me she was convinced of its value. My friend had a hysterectomy in her early thirties as a treatment for cancer and now took hormones daily herself.

The conversation returned to the incest. It was possible that my lack of periods was due to my amnesia ending and my experience of trauma. The brain can do tricks.

"When did it start?" Robin asked, referring to the abuse.

"I don't even think I was one. My earliest memory is being on a white table. I think I was still in diapers, maybe it was a bassinet. I'm not sure. A man hit me really hard in the crotch and I cried. It's not completely clear. Later I was forced to give him oral sex. It went on for years."

She had heard stories like this before. I continued, "when I was living in Maine, it seemed like there were a lot of incest survivors. Now I'm in New York City and I don't know any. None of my friends are."

"That is hard to believe," said Robin. "It seems like the women I see are all survivors."

I felt myself shaking inside. The conversation stirred up so many emotions. I mentioned that I had been in therapy in Maine until our move in late August. Now I was looking for a therapist in New York. She gave me two names. I started crying and grabbed some tissues from the box on her desk.

"I feel like such a downer, such a burden to my friends. I never seem to have any good news. First it's cancer, then it's cancer again, and now it's incest." I collapsed into sobs. "I just want to be well and happy."

"That is self hate," Robin said.

"I know. I figured that out last week."

"You need more than your friends. They cannot truly understand what you are going through. You have been through a lot and you are strong and brave. You will get through this too. You have opened yourself to it and now you must go through the process. It's not going to be easy. Sometimes you won't want to go on but you will. You CAN heal. Once you get through this you will have a whole new life. It may take a long time. You can't rush healing."

I listened to her. I tried to take it all in. Healing seemed so far away, so unreachable. She convinced me she had seen people progress through healing, and I left her office with hope.

Changes: The Before and the After

Beverly Lickteig Loder

Three years ago last August, the colors changed. Some may gently protest, attempt to dissuade me from this observation, but I am here to tell you that without a doubt, the colors changed.

It happened as I fled the first floor of Elmhurst Clinic, sailing past anonymous nurses and distracted patients, wondering if I looked somehow different to them, like a person who had just been diagnosed with a dread disease. *I* certainly hadn't recognized the woman who had looked back at me from the mirror in the small examining room, the woman with the profound fear in her eyes.

The doctor's words echoed in my ears, "Our worst suspicions have been confirmed. . . ." I knew my face would never look quite the same to me again, and this knowledge has become truth. I was twenty-nine years old and I had breast cancer. For me, it was the end of the innocence.

It was one of those glorious late summer days when God's light shines down golden as cornsilk, lending a burnished glow to sloping sidewalks and straight-shot highways. Stepping out into the unnatural brightness, I joined the ranks of poets who have railed against the graceless sun, who have fervently wished it would rain.

As I drove the eight miles to my parents' home, I turned on my radio, hoping that the familiar voice of the deejay would cut through this surreal feeling, return me to some sensible place. But the realization that the world was calmly going on without me made me feel more desperately unnerved than ever.

I found myself letting out a long, terrified cry of pure anguish.

Later, I perched alone on the patio steps in the backyard of my childhood home. It was the first silence to permeate the shock, the sliding glass door a transparent shield against the horror I had dumped onto the kitchen floor at my mother's feet. For the moment, I had to block out the steadily rising rallying cry of my family as the news spread from person to person, my cancer infiltrating their lives as surely as mine.

I couldn't face their reactions: the disbelief in my sisters' voices, the unspeakable grief and rage in my mother's eyes as she raised her fist to pound heaven, the heartwrenching poignancy of one brother's inability to look at me at all. And my little girl, happily playing with the neighborhood kids down the block, oblivious to any threat to her secure routine—what would she think? How could I convince her that we would still live happily ever after, together forever?

And so I came face to face with my own mortality, gazing out at the place most familiar to my eyes— the lush, green grass and overflowing beds of brilliantly hued blossoms, the result of my father's hard sweat and labor and his Kansas farmboy magic. I remembered all the endless summers I spent out here in this magical haven, rolling down the sloped lawn as a child, catching lightning bugs in the twilight. These trees and flowers served as backdrop to hundreds of photographs over the years; the flowering crabtrees framed prom and graduation portraits, the marigolds formed bright halos around the heads of laughing children and grandchildren. As I let the memories wash over me in waves, I wondered how many more summers I had left to look out on this, my childhood refuge.

Although this was a scene I had looked out on endlessly over twenty-five years of my life, now it seemed different. The glorious reds, greens, golds, and violets were unnaturally bright. And the colors had changed.

But the colors aren't all that have changed. I have changed, too, in subtle ways that nudge me only now and then; in deeper, unfathomable ways that have altered my outlook for all time. Sometimes I come across photographs of me taken several years back. Reflexively I think, "I didn't have cancer then. I didn't *know*." And I scrutinize my face in the picture, searching my eyes for that glint of innocence I know I will never recapture. I try to recall the way I felt the day the photo was snapped—the invincibility, the fearlessness of youth. I doubt I would trade the knowledge I've gained from my experience for my former naivete, but there are times when I think it would be blissful ignorance to forget, even for one day, that I ever had cancer.

Not that I obsess on the fact; I don't. When I was going through the surgeries and the treatments, it was almost impossible to put aside: I couldn't block out the thought of cancer when my body was being ravaged by "cures" far more painful than the symptoms of the disease. With the passing of time, I have healed in both body and mind, and the fear of recurrence, although omnipresent, has been relegated to the ranks of any human fear. It's there, but it's manageable. Cancer is a vivid, striking piece of my past. It has influenced the way I perceive life, but it is in my *past* and it does not control me.

I have accepted that this unspeakable thing has happened and have acknowledged that it can come back. But I draw great comfort from the truth that I beat it once and have every faith that I could beat it again. Recurrence is undoubtedly the biggest fear of former cancer patients, particularly with a disease that no doctor can promise you is gone forever. We do well to confront this fear and keep it in perspective. Some people say anyone can go out and get hit by a truck—that we're all equally at risk. What those people don't understand is that some of us have already been hit by that truck and wonder whether it's circling the block.

As I child, I was a skinny little thing, but no one dared call me fragile. I saw myself as tough and strong, and held my own in neighborhood kickball games and in wrestling with my brothers. Although painfully sensitive, I never wanted to be perceived as weak. I could take care of myself. That independence made it tough to accept a diagnosis of cancer. I didn't want anyone to feel sorry for me, least of all people who didn't even know me.

After chemotherapy, I joined a support group for women with breast cancer. In the beginning it was a great relief to talk with other women who'd fought the same battles. I was amazed at what similar experiences such a disparate group of women could have. We were young and old, married and divorced, with and without children. I was struck by the incredible fortitude displayed by these quiet, polite women. As one of them noted, my perception of what constitutes the heroes of this world has been completely resketched.

The support group provided a forum where no subject was taboo. Everybody's fears and dark nightmares were thrown on the table for discussion. For a time, I found the group helpful and therapeutic. Eventually I noticed I was leaving sessions feeling anxious and depressed. It became draining for me to share so much with these people; I was no longer taking anything positive away. It became painful to hear of the recurrences some group members were experiencing. It was time to move on.

The support group was a good interim step for me following my treatments. We all felt somehow safe in our circle; we shared one hard-learned truth. I was pleased to be able to share advice, hoping I could help another. But I also found myself looking at the faces around me and wondering who would survive and who would die. After a while, I needed to get past that one common bond.

Now when I meet people, I do not immediately tell them of my experience with cancer. Shortly after my diagnosis, it was hard to avoid the subject. Now I may not tell acquaintances at all. It may eventually emerge from a conversation about the book I am writing or the volunteer work I do for the American Cancer Society. Cancer is not now a focus in my life, though, and it's just not necessary to bring up the subject as it was when I was in crisis.

I began a new job just weeks after my mastectomy. Although only a few coworkers had prior knowledge of my illness when I started that job, only a short time passed before all the twenty-odd people in my close-knit department were aware of my condition. Most were sympathetic and kind. But this wasn't quite what I'd hoped for in starting a new job: I wanted to be judged on the merits of my skills, befriended for who I was, not because I was the young editor with cancer, poor soul. Eventually, people related to me the way I wanted, but it took longer to form friendships with them because I was wary of their perceptions of me.

An important development for me has been that I *can* talk about my cancer experience with ease if I want to. It took me a good year after chemotherapy to get to that place; before that, it was uncomfortable to discuss. A small, irrational part of me thought that if I talked about it too much, it would come back—that fear of recurrence might become a self-fulfilling prophecy.

But you can't stay afraid forever. We all have stress. When my anxiety level peaks, I've learned to take a moment and let go. I don't think about the problem at hand, and I don't think about cancer. In fact, not too much throws me anymore. Permanently losing a breast has something to do with that. Temporarily losing all my hair and much of my self-esteem changed my attitude as well. I figure if I could come through the atrocities of chemotherapy, I can probably make it through that unexpected crisis that just landed on my desk at work. Ask anyone who's survived it: Cancer makes you stronger. Overcome your fear and turn your apprehension into a fierce will to live, and you discover an amazing depth of spirit within. Turn this drive to positive growth and there's no limit to the heights you'll climb.

One of the challenges is adjusting to a sudden shift in body image. Many of us gain or lose weight, but without cancer it doesn't usually happen all at once. Wrinkles and gray hair creep up on us, gradually. We get used to the changes in the mirror when they occur over time. Once when I was depressed about the loss of my breast, a close friend admonished me not to be so vain. He said that when his hairline began receding when he was only in his twenties, nobody cared but his mother. I was quick to point out that he hadn't awoken one morning to find all his hair on his pillow—he hadn't gone bald overnight. Besides, I pointed out, it's not vain to prefer a breast to a raging red slash across your chest, once-soft skin now stretched over your heart as tightly as a drum.

My scars are no longer quite so jarring. Reconstructive surgery provided some camouflage, and the skin has grown soft again. The scars themselves are less prominent, coexisting benignly with the healthy skin surrounding them, almost blending in. The angry red has faded to a pale, silvery pink. The colors have changed. They're not necessarily better or worse. But they are different.

My prior cancer status deems me both saint and renegade. I have a bad habit of unconsciously dividing my friends and colleagues into those who knew me "before" and those who have only known me "after." It seems a curious division, but there is something precious to me about those who remember who I was before. They remember how I always took that unbeaten path—first to fall in love, first to move away from home, first to marry, give birth, divorce. Always taking the hard road, but somehow emerging with a smile, much wiser though slightly battered from the journey. I survived a tumultuous early marriage to a drug abuser and several lean years while I struggled to simultaneously work, raise my child, and finish my degree. I came to believe there was no obstacle I couldn't overcome with hard work and heartfelt prayers. Of course, I didn't count on having to tackle cancer. Nobody ever does.

CAUTION:
IVF May Be Harmful to Your Health

Rita Arditti

Gilda Radner, a TV star, a woman who loved to make people laugh, famous for her appearances on *Saturday Night Live*, was diagnosed with ovarian cancer in October 1986 and died in early 1989. In her autobiography, *It's Always Something*, she writes with great honesty and openness about her anxieties as a TV star, her ambition to become a movie star, her eating disorders, and her love for her husband. "It's always something" was her father's favorite expression and an appropriate title for Radner's story. The book became a bestseller in 1989 and was released in paperback in 1990.

Radner begins the book with a description of her wedding in southern France in 1984 to Gene Wilder, also a comedian, and her joy at the prospect of having children and building a life with him. Soon after the marriage, however, she learned that she was infertile and that in order to conceive she would have to have major surgery to open her blocked Fallopian tubes, or go through *in vitro* fertilization. She enrolled in the *in vitro* fertilization program at UCLA and, inspired by the enthusiasm of the *in vitro* team, went through the procedure faithfully.

At this point in reading the book, my antennae went up: might there have been some connection between the daily hormone treatments that Radner received during IVF and her subsequent development of ovarian cancer? A number of reported cases

exist of cancer growing after clomiphene treatment.[*]
A 1977 article reports two cases of breast cancer associated with clomiphene.[**] A more recent paper
describes a case of rapidly growing ovarian cancer
in a woman on an IVF program who took clomiphene followed by HMG (human menopausal
gonadotrophin) and HCG (human chorionic
gonadotrophin).[***] Additionally, the authors cite two
previous cases in which ovarian cancer followed ovulation induction, and they cite a paper suggesting
that elevated gonadotrophin levels are implicated in
the development of ovarian tumors.[+] Though the
hormones may not directly initiate tumor formation,
they can act to promote carcinogenesis.

Describing the IVF procedure in simple and clear
terms, Radner acknowledges that, although it was
"horrible," she was willing to repeat the procedure
if it did not work the first time. The superovulatory
treatment produced eight eggs, seven of which were
fertilized in a Petri dish. Four fertilized eggs were
implanted in her uterus, and three were thrown
away. After the implantation she continued to
receive hormone injections. Even after she started to
bleed and knew that she was miscarrying, her doctors insisted on continuing the shots, because it "was
an experimental procedure and they had to follow
their protocol." Of course, she was right; she did not
get pregnant.

As she put it, "my ovaries became the center of
my universe." She also underwent major surgery to
have her tubes opened. She did eventually get preg-

---

[*] Clomiphene citrate is a drug commonly used in infertility
treatment and on IVF programs, see Klein and Rowland, 1988.

[**] Bolton, 1977.

[***] Carter and Joyce, 1987.

[+] Cramer and Welch, 1983.

nant, but she miscarried and then threw herself into work, thinking that she would have children later on.

Radner tells the history of cancer in her family. Her father died of a malignant brain tumor, but it is on her mother's side of the family that cancer was very much a factor. Her mother's mother died of stomach cancer, Gilda's mother has had metastatic breast cancer, her mother's sister also died of stomach cancer, and that aunt's youngest daughter has had cancer in both breasts and in her ovaries. It is likely that the "stomach cancer" of her grandmother and of her aunt was really ovarian cancer; cancer of the ovaries produces symptoms sometimes attributed to stomach trouble. In fact, in her long and futile search to alleviate her pain in the abdominal area, Radner was told that she had a stomach problem.

With a family history like this, why was Radner accepted in a program that involved hormonal treatments that would most likely increase her chances of getting cancer?

Radner's case demonstrates the low regard of the medical establishment for women's lives, as it takes advantage of women's vulnerability to "help women get pregnant at any cost." Do the proliferating *in vitro* programs around the world take into account the histories of cancer in women's families? Do they even suggest to a woman that it may be harmful for her to take superovulatory hormones? Is anyone doing long-term follow-up studies on the thousands of women who have gone through these programs, to see whether their cancer rates are higher than normal? Does anybody care?

A November 1989 pamphlet published by the American Fertility Society entitled "Questions to Ask about an IVF/Gift program" does not list one single question about the short- or long-term consequences of IVF for the woman's health and well-being. The pamphlet's 30 suggested questions deal with success rates, details about the program, and financial issues. Reading it gives one the impression that IVF/Gift, highly invasive and interventionistic procedures, do not take place in women's bodies but in some remote, non-human site.

In discussing what may have been the factors that contributed to her developing ovarian cancer, Radner mentions smoking, wrong foods, red candies, barbecues, etc. As she put it, "Whatever the American Cancer Society says causes cancer, I have undoubtedly done it." *It's Always Something* contains not one word about the hormones that were used to stimulate her ovaries during her IVF. Radner was more than willing to take responsibility for her behavior and to acknowledge that she may have contributed to her cancer. But how possible is to conduct a life that will make one totally "cancer-immune"? We do a real disservice to all of us if we focus this way on personal behavior and lose track of the bigger picture. "Blaming the victim" is a handy response to the cancer epidemic in the United States, where one out of three women will develop cancer at some time in her life. This mentality individualizes health problems and reduces all to "personal" responsibility. Where is the responsibility of the health care system that lets a woman with a family cancer history like Gilda Radner's enter a program in which hormonal manipulations are paramount?

Before Radner's cancer diagnosis, she went through a long period of not feeling well and having all kinds of symptoms. Because her medical tests looked okay, she was told that her problems were "emotional." With great sense of humor she called herself "The Queen of Neurosis." No wonder she felt relieved when they did find a malignancy—then there was a chance that she could finally get some help. Just as had happened to her father, Radner went through the diagnosis and initial treatment with nobody ever saying the word *cancer*. She had a total hysterectomy but did not realize until *after* the operation that her reproductive organs had been removed. So much for "informed consent" and successful doctor-patient communication.

Gilda Radner found companionship and solace in the Wellness Community, a group in Santa Monica, California, where cancer patients meet, share their experiences, and support each other to make their lives better. She learned to do visualization, guided imagery, and relaxation to reduce the stress that her condition brought into her life. She invented funny little songs to keep her spirits up. As her condition worsened, Radner tried macrobiotics and wore all-cotton clothes, trying to live a more balanced, more natural life. Though the cancer did not go away, she used the process as another learning experience to deepen her understanding of her own attitudes and beliefs.

I do not know whether all the painful treatments Radner endured extended her life at all, or if she would have lived just as long (or as short) had she stopped after her initial treatment. Her story also points out that overreliance on technology can have very negative effects on people's lives. For example, due to a computer error, Radner received misinformation about her condition. As a result, she was totally unprepared for the cancer's recurrence, which was diagnosed when she changed doctors.

That a woman like Radner, with so many personal connections and financial resources, went through the pain and hell she did, reveals the sorry state of current medical cancer treatments and the urgency of opening the field of cancer research to much-needed new ideas. Her story is one more addition to the growing list of abuses perpetrated on women's bodies in the name of scientific and technological "progress."

REFERENCES

Bolton, P.M. "Bilateral Breast Cancer Associated with Clomiphene." The Lancet, 3 December 1977: 1176.

Carter, Marian E. and Joyce, David N. "Ovarian Carcinoma in a Patient Hyperstimulated by Gonadotropin Therapy for In Vitro Fertilization: A Case Report." Journal of In Vitro Fertilization and Embryo Transfer 4(2): 126–128. 1987.

Cramer, Daniel W. and Welch, William R. "Determinants of Ovarian Cancer Risk. II. Inferences Regarding Pathogenesis." Journal of the National Cancer Institute 71(4): 717–721. 1983.

Klein, Renate and Rowland, Robyn. "Women as Test-sites for Fertility Drugs: Clomiphene Citrate and Hormonal Cocktails." Reproductive and Genetic Engineering 1 (3): 251–273. 1988.

Radner, Gilda. It's Always Something. New York: Simon and Schuster, 1989. (Paperback edition by Avon Books, New York, 1990.)

Lifestyles Don't Kill.
Carcinogens in Air, Food, and Water Do.
Imagining Political Responses to Cancer

Sandra Steingraber

Summer 1990 in Chicago, great public fuss was
generated by the short-lived appearance of an AIDS
poster in subways and buses. Promoted by ACT-UP
as a public service announcement and narrowly
approved after much grandstanding and speechify-
ing at the Illinois State House, the poster called for a
political understanding of AIDS and an end to vic-
tim-blaming attitudes. "Kissing doesn't kill. Greed
and Indifference Do." The words framed images of
three young couples kissing—two women, two men,
and an interracial male/female couple. Near the bottom, the smaller print explained, "Corporate greed,
government inaction, and public indifference make
AIDS a political crisis."

Interestingly, it was the pictures and not the
words that provoked the most controversy. Fears
that gay-positive imagery would "promote" a gay
lifestyle were at the center of the objections. A few
newspaper columnists and writers to the editor wondered if the message was overly cryptic. But for the
most part, the assumption that AIDS has political as
well as biological roots was not questioned. After a
one-month run, with various attendant threats of
defacement, the posters vanished.

As a cancer activist,[*] I was both heartened and

---

[*] My personal evolution toward activism is described in the essay
"We All Live Downwind," in *The Women and Cancer Anthology*,
ed. J. Brady (Pittsburgh, PA: Cleis Press, fall 1991).

91

dismayed by this little drama. On the one hand, the public reaction against the photos revealed the deep currents of homophobia that still run just under the surface of public concern about AIDS. On the other hand, I was reminded that the public debate about cancer almost never approaches the same open acknowledgement of the disease's social causes and contexts that discussions of AIDS do. Discussions about AIDS—even in confrontational settings—can seem downright enlightened compared to discussions about cancer. There is a kind of public silence surrounding cancer: sadness but not outrage, fearful awareness but not confrontation, victims but not street warriors, private suspicions but not political action.

There are undoubtedly several reasons for this silence and the difference between how we think about AIDS and how we think about cancer. First, with AIDS the issue of contagion has forced us to speak clearly about risk factors and prevention. This attention has laid bare the social, political, and economic roots in a way that has never really happened with cancer, a disease with many and uncertain causes. Second, few easily identifiable communities of people exist to champion a campaign around cancer. Third, cancer has two very conservative and powerful research and medical establishments, the American Cancer Society (ACS) and the National Cancer Institute (NCI), that shape public perception and education almost completely and have very skillfully depoliticized the issues. The apolitical representation of cancer by the ACS and the NCI present a formidable challenge to grassroots groups with more radical analyses.*

What would meaningful political responses to cancer look like? We could start by being clear about the death toll. One in three women will be diagnosed with cancer sometime during her life. About half of those—or one in every six of us—will die. The statistics reveal our immense vulnerability. Imagine what a quilt embroidered with the names of the cancer dead would look like.

Yet our ostensible cancer advocacy organizations use these same statistics to erase us. An NCI pamphlet recently disseminated at a Northwestern Memorial Hospital forum about cancer, part of a series of lectures on health issues for women, begins its cheery message under the pink and blue heading, "Good News: Everyone does not get cancer. 2 out of 3 Americans will never get it." Under this banner is another even more misleading proclamation: "Better News: Every year more and more people with cancer are cured."

What is not said, of course, is that the cure RATE has hardly changed at all. As the incidence rate rises, the numbers of both the cured and the non-

---

* These include the Women's Community Cancer Project in Boston, the Mautner Project for Lesbians with Cancer in Washington, D.C., the Lesbian Community Cancer Project in Chicago, and the Women's Cancer Resource Center in Oakland. The work and writing of feminist author Susan Shapiro has been tremendously inspirational in the founding of the grassroots cancer groups for women. Before her death in 1990, Shapiro called for a feminist response to cancer: "Cancer is clearly a feminist issue. We need an organization—of women, for women—that will encompass political action, direct service, and education" (from "Cancer as a Feminist Issue," *Sojourner*, September 1989).

cured go up. What is not said is that more people are also dying of cancer every year.

This pamphlet is typical of the slick and colorful messages that go out to school health classes, doctor's offices, libraries, clinics, etc. These are the words that shape public perception.

It is not clear to me why the public education programs of the ACS and the NCI choose to minimize the casualties. By the NCI's own findings, the breast cancer incidence rate alone increased by 32 percent in the past decade.* Overall cancer mortality among those over 55 has risen steeply and steadily over the past two decades.** The incidence of childhood cancer has risen 22 percent since 1950.*** Perhaps false optimism and the implication of constant progress and imminent breakthroughs ("we are winning") make fundraising easier. I do know for sure that many of us struggling with cancer and cancer histories feel isolated and invisible in the face of winning-the-war propaganda.

And I do know that members of the medical community very often perpetuate and reinforce the rhetoric. At that same Northwestern cancer forum, for example, gynecologic oncologist Julian Schink actually stood at a podium, looked out at the women in the auditorium, smiled and said, "You need to keep breast cancer in perspective....More women die each year by falling and breaking their

---

  * Cited in Jane Gross, "Turning Breast Cancer into a Cause: Breast Cancer Follows AIDS," *New York Times* (Jan. 7, 1990), p. A1, col. 1; and Claudia Wallis, "A Puzzling Plague: What is it About the American Way of Life that Causes Breast Cancer?" *Time* (Jan. 14, 1991), pp. 48–52.

 ** Natalie Angier, "Cancer Rates Rising Steeply for Those 55 or Older," *New York Times* (Aug. 24, 1990).

*** National Cancer Institute, cited in Harper's Index, *Harper's*, March 1990, p. 19.

hips than die of breast cancer." I sat there quietly, thinking first, "well, that's a lot of dead women," and then, "HE DOESN'T CARE ABOUT US." The entire auditorium was silent—maybe stunned—but silent nevertheless. No one in the audience confronted him. No one walked out. I can't imagine that any doctor could tell an audience of people with AIDS to keep their disease in perspective and be met with such complicity.

▲ ▲ ▲

We need a public education campaign that embraces the facts and rings the alarm bell. Like ACT-UP, we need to stand up and take charge. We need to count the living and the dead and post the numbers publicly. We need to make it known that we ARE the one third who are struggling with cancer. We need to make it known that we as women are also the prime caretakers of others with cancer, that we as women are too poor and too busy to continue quietly dying and taking care of the dead and dying, that we as women find a 32-percent increase in breast cancer incidence unacceptable, and that we are thus outraged and demand change. We can start by replacing the "Good News" banner with one that reads "Yes, it is really THAT BAD."

The feminist grassroots cancer movement now forming is indeed doing much toward this new accounting. Jackie Winnow of the Women's Cancer Resource Center in Oakland, for example, puts cancer "in perspective" with the following comparison:

> In 1988, approximately forty thousand women were living with cancer in the San Francisco/Oakland area, at least four thousand being lesbians, about four thousand women dying. The forty thousand women don't have the services that the hun-

dred women with AIDS have. I want the women
with AIDS to have these services. I don't mean to
polarize. But I also want recognition that we have a
huge problem here and we need to do something
about it.[*]

As the grassroots movement grows and we
become more visible and more vocal, the issue of
identity politics arises. What do we call ourselves?
With what identities do we experience and understand this disease? Are we cancer victims? cancer
survivors? cancer patients? people with cancer?
women with cancer? feminists with cancer? lesbians
with cancer? These were the questions a group of us
addressed at the Audre Lorde "I Am Your Sister"
celeconference in Boston in October 1990. The tense
question is also a tricky one: when exactly *do* we or
did we have cancer? For those with systemic or
metastasized cancer, having cancer becomes its own
ongoing and present-tense identity. Others of us prefer the optimism of the past tense: we "had cancer"
between diagnosis and surgery, and now (we hope)
the experience is past. Even while undergoing post-
surgical chemotherapy or radiation treatment, we
presume we are now cancer-free and conceptualize
the ongoing torment as a preventative measure, a
mop-up operation, a kind of insurance against
future malignancy.

Or should all of us, like those who are now speaking out about incest, refer to ourselves as cancer
"survivors"? Some find the term empowering. Others—myself included—feel the term divides us in
half (and who wants to be in the other half?) and at
the same time denies the uncertainty of our progno-

---

[*] Jackie Winnow, "Lesbians Evolving Health Care: Our Lives
Depend on It," *Sinister Wisdom 39* (1989), p. 53; also this
volume, p. 25.

sis, one of the major issues with which we have to struggle. The Boston-based Women's Community Cancer Project has settled on the slightly cumbersome but inclusive term "women with cancer and cancer histories." This term was also adopted by the Lesbian Community Cancer Project in Chicago.

Strong positive feelings and negative feelings exist about the term "cancer victim." Journalist and cancer advocate Jory Graham preached against its usage on the grounds that the word "victim" objectifies those living with cancer, insinuates helplessness, and supersedes personhood and achievement.[*]

Writer and editor Judy Brady, in contrast, uses the term "cancer victim" to great effect.[**] She argues that cancer IS a victimizing, objectifying experience which euphemisms cannot and should not erase. I myself use the term when I want to highlight the notion that cancer is both a preventable disease and a human rights issue.

As a biologist, I am convinced that the growing incidence of cancer in our communities is a direct consequence of behavior on the part of government and industry that violates our right to a safe environment. By identifying as "victims," we ally ourselves with women who have experienced other forms of criminal victimization (by rape, battery, crime, harassment, discrimination, etc.) and can empower ourselves by working toward social change. From this position, we can call for comprehensive legislation to prevent and punish victimization by

---

[*] Jory Graham, *In the Company of Others: Understanding the Human Needs of Cancer Patients* (New York: Harcourt Brace Jovanowich, 1982), pp. 133–135.

[**] Brady, Judy, "The Goose and the Golden Egg," in *The Women and Cancer Anthology*, op. cit.

environmental poisoning, thus dramatically reducing the incidence of cancer.

▲ ▲ ▲

The issue of prevention should absolutely rank at
the top of our agenda of political responses to cancer. Addressing prevention in a meaningful way is
probably the most daunting task we have—and the
most threatening. As Judy Brady points out, a campaign of real cancer prevention—unlike AIDS
prevention work—would have to challenge the
whole political and economic structure of industrial
capitalism. Jackie Winnow has also spoken clearly
about this: "Actual prevention would mean changing society—cleaning it up....Everyone knows that
pollution causes cancer, but does the NCI or the
American Cancer Society do anything about it?"*
Audre Lorde urges us to replace New Age heal-
thyself concepts of disease prevention with political
action: "It is easier to demand happiness than clean
up the environment....The idea that happiness can
insulate us against the results of our environmental
madness is a rumor circulated by our enemies to
destroy us."** Indeed.

Amazingly, it is possible to read entire public educational tracts about cancer published by the ACS
and the NCI without ever encountering the idea that
cancers are caused by carcinogens. For example, the
NCI "Good News" brochure given to all of us at the
Northwestern forum refers frequently to "risk factors" and contains a list of "cancer prevention tips."
These include staying out of the sun, limiting alco-
hol consumption, eating high fiber foods, not

---

*   Winnow, op. cit.

** Audre Lorde, *The Cancer Journals* (San Francisco: Spinsters/Aunt
     Lute, 1980), pp. 74–75.

smoking, avoiding "unnecessary x-rays" (whatever those are), and obeying the "health and safety rules of your workplace." Then follows a detailed explanation of the role of dietary fiber in reducing "risk."[*]

Not only do the ACS and the NCI fail to help us understand how personal habits are themselves social constructions, but the lifestyle emphasis also obscures the role of environmental hazards that are beyond personal choice. By referring to "risks," rather than "carcinogens," these seemingly authoritative agencies frame the cause of the disease as a problem of *behavior* (risky or non-risky) rather than as a problem of *exposure* to disease-causing agents. We have to start asking questions about what the lifestyle approach to cancer leaves out. The "Good News" cancer brochure does not mention the study by the International Commission on Radiological Protection that concludes that cancer risk from ionizing radiation (x-rays, radon, nuclear power plants) is about three times higher than believed previously.[**] It does not mention the U.S. government's admission that it covered up evidence of high rates of cancer among workers in the Hanford nuclear weapons plant and among downwind residents.[***] It does not mention a study released by the National Safe Workplace Institute identifying cancer as the

---

[*] In "We All Live Downwind," *The Women and Cancer Anthology* (Cleis Press, fall 1991), I examine in detail the fixation on personal lifestyle in the public educational campaigns of the ACS and the NCI.

[**] Cited in "Cut Maximum Allowable Radiation Dose, Panel Recommends," *Chicago Tribune* (June 24, 1990), sec. 1, p. 20.

[***] "World Shocker: Scientist Who Warned of Peril to Atomic Workers," *Chicago Tribune* (June 24, 1990), sec. 6, p. 4; Keith Schneider, "U.S. Sees a Danger in 1940s Radiation in the Northwest," *New York Times* (July 12, 1990), p. A1; and Tom Bailie, "Growing Up as a Nuclear Guinea Pig," *New York Times* (July 22, 1990), p. A19.

number one occupational-disease killer—responsible for at least 24,000 deaths every year.* It does not mention that well-documented cancer clusters have been mapped in communities located near chemical factories, refineries, nuclear reactors, and pesticide-laden farm fields.** It does not mention Love Canal, Times Beach, Minamata, Chernobyl, Three Mile Island, or Bhopal.

▲ ▲ ▲

Those of us doing cancer activist work also have to become better medical research watchdogs. If AIDS activists can figure out the ins and outs of virology and drug-testing, we can start monitoring why certain kinds of cancer studies get funding and media coverage and others do not. And we can lobby for what we want answers to. For example, I am nearly convinced that the great emphasis on genetic factors in predisposing us to cancer has more to do with the ease and appeal of doing that kind of science than it does in explaining accelerating cancer rates. To assess our cancer risk, doctors routinely ask us if our mothers or sisters have had cancer. They do not ask us if we grew up near a toxic waste dump or a garbage incinerator.

Does this imply that doctors blame women for their own diseases? Maybe or maybe not. Do we find it more comfortable to blame our mothers than to find out what pesticides are in the food supply? Perhaps. But we should not conclude that the constant emphasis on family history means that what's in our genes is more important than what's in our

---

* Merrill Goozner, "Job Diseases Remain a Major Cause of Death," *Chicago Tribune* (Aug. 31, 1990), sec. 1, p. 1.

** Richard Swift, "Breaking the Grip of Cancer," *The New Internationalist 198* (August 1989), p. 4.

drinking water. More likely, the studies that would establish an environmental link have never been done. Most women who have been diagnosed with breast cancer, for example, have no family history of the disease at all.

Before we can ask others to divest themselves of cancer stigmas and myths, we have to educate ourselves and question our own assumptions about the disease. We then need to demand answers from the medical research community. For example, is a diet high in animal fat really linked to breast cancer? If so, is that because of the fat itself or because of carcinogens concentrated in the fat of the animals we eat? Those studies haven't been done yet? Why not? Women are dying; we need to know now.

▲ ▲ ▲

As we develop our political responses to the cancer crisis, alliances and divisions will undoubtedly form. Grassroots environmental groups, particularly the anti-toxics organizations, have accumulated a wealth of information about cancer rates in different communities as well as having wily political skills. Family farm organizations monitor all manner of research on the health effects of various agricultural chemicals—a coalition of farm and consumer groups, for example, is currently spearheading the opposition to a synthetic hormone (BGH) in the milk supply. Civil rights groups are beginning to look at toxic dumping in inner city areas. All of these groups would be potential allies to a feminist cancer movement and are often repositories of hard-to-find studies and reports.

I am somewhat concerned by the potential split between lesbians and non-lesbians. Already, two of the groups, the Mautner Project in Washington D.C.

and the Lesbian Community Cancer Project in Chicago, have focused their energy on forming support networks and direct services for women in the lesbian community. Many of their volunteers bring considerable experience and insight from working in the AIDS service community and seek to replicate similar structures of support for lesbians with cancer in their own communities. An outsider to the lesbian community, I do understand and respect the need for a lesbian-centered support and care system. I certainly believe that our experience of illness is inscribed by all of our particular identities.

But I hope we can do more than learn to be caregivers—of whatever kind—to the sick and dying. I also know with every cell in my body that the political crisis of cancer is a feminist issue—from television ads for diet products to mammograms, from health insurance travesties to impoverished single mothers living in toxics-riddled neighborhoods—and that only a unified and orchestrated response from within the women's movement can begin to address it. We must take what has victimized us and turn it into a force of political change.

As I write, radio commentators are discussing the high-stakes practice of bombing Iraqi nuclear power plants, setting new precedents for warfare. I learn that Baghdad is a city of four million people, most of whom are women and children. Over Iran, downwind of torched oil fields, a black oily rain is falling. Those of us who have lived through the hell of cancer diagnosis and treatment should be expressing public outrage. The ACS and the NCI will never add "bombing nuclear sites" to their list of "risky behaviors." We have to. Or perhaps we could simply start with a few posters in the subway: "Lifestyles don't kill. Carcinogens in air, food and water do."

One Day At a Time:

Excerpts from a Journal

Rita Arditti

In 1974 I found a lump in my breast that turned out to be malignant. I was 39 years old. I had an operation that removed my right breast and 18 lymph nodes, followed by 21 radiation treatments. I was well for four years, then I started developing a cough that resisted all treatments, and by 1979 I was diagnosed as having metastatic cancer in my lungs. What follows are excerpts from my journal from 1974 through 1984.

1974

May 18—I told Dr. Kennan that I felt a lump in my breast. He could not find it and for a moment I thought I would leave the examining table without a lump any more. But I insisted, and since he still could not find it, I took his hand and put it right over the lump. Now he agreed, yes, there was something there.

May 23—Dr. Resnick immediately said that this looks "serious," and I did not like the look on his face. He called the surgeon, Dr. Frazier, and they wanted me to go into the hospital as soon as possible and agree to a modified radical mastectomy if the lump is cancerous. The way they put it, I would go into the operating room and not know if I would wake up with one breast or two. I could not believe it. I said that I needed time to think about this, and Dr. Resnick got angry with me. He warned that I was playing with my life. Dr. Frazier did not say

103

much, but he looked more reasonable. What scares me most is the general anesthesia. Countless stories in my childhood of people not "waking up" from it. I feel strangely calm and distant as if this whole thing is not happening to me. I never thought I would get cancer. There is no cancer in my family. Right now I feel very tired and I would love a warm body to cuddle against. But there is no one here.

May 24—Dr. Frazier is okay. After I said there was no way that I would agree to a mastectomy without first knowing, fully awake, that the lump is cancer, he came up with a new idea. He will do a needle biopsy, remove a little bit of the tissue and see what is there. Of course, if the result is negative then we have to do a lumpectomy, remove the whole lump and check it carefully. If it is positive, then he will do the mastectomy. If I need the operation, he says it will take four to six days in the hospital and about two weeks recovery with excellent recovery foreseeable.

I know I have to write my family and my son's father, but I do not have the strength right now. I asked Dr. Frazier if I should write a will and he shook his head. He said it was not appropriate at this time. Either one has a will because one is prepared (and everyone should be) or one does it later. A will should not be done in a moment of crisis.

Today I got a really good letter from my mother. I hate to tell her about my bad news.

June 1—Dr. Frazier's secretary held my hand while he did the biopsy. It did not hurt that much. I had local anesthesia. I went out to dinner and had three Bloody Marys and a plush supper.

June 4—It's carcinoma. No doubt about it. Dr. Frazier told me over the phone "We both know what the result is." He says for a lesion this size the only thing he is comfortable doing is a modified radical. I want to live.

June 5—Before I decide on the mastectomy, I want to hear what the "other side" says. Dr. Clay does not do mastectomies. He takes the lump out and after studying it carefully, he suggests a treatment which could be radiation, chemotherapy, or further surgery. I saw him today, and indeed, he said he would not do a mastectomy. I am feeling quite crazy. My friend Rena suggested I get a third-party opinion. I made an appointment to see Dr. Mitchell, supposedly a great authority on all this.

June 6—Dr. Mitchell is the fatherly kind, but he was quite blunt; he thinks Dr. Clay is senile, and he said that radiologists do not even know if radiation can kill cancer cells. He added that he would not let anyone in his family get the sort of treatment Dr. Clay proposes. He ended up saying that Dr. Frazier is an excellent doctor and I should trust him, adding somewhat dramatically, "Frazier has been in Vietnam, he knows about life and death." He said I was unlucky to be caught in 1974 with this problem: two years ago nobody would have challenged a mastectomy, and two years from now we may know about the new therapies. But this is the moment of transition and uncertainty. He was angry that the media had given so much attention to the criticisms of breast cancer treatment and said that, in his view, Dr. Clay was the worst of them all. I am strangely relieved. I may be railroaded, but he sounded right to me. I will have the mastectomy.[*]

The good news is that my sister Edith is here. She arrived yesterday morning from Argentina. Her plane had a difficult landing; it seemed that the wheels were not coming out, and there were fire-trucks and ambulances waiting for the plane. We laughed about it. Here she came to help me with my cancer and her own life is endangered!

June 7—I called Dr. Frazier and told him I was ready. He snapped back, "Ready for what?" I said, "For the operation, you know..." I said I had to do it my way. Before I was not ready for it. Now I am. He seemed to understand and even added that in my place, he might have done the same. He wanted me to show up at the hospital right away, but I told him my son was graduating from elementary school and that I had promised to go to the graduation ceremony at eleven, so that I would get to the hospital around two or three o'clock.

The operation will be tomorrow morning. I do not know if I will be able to write in my journal after-ward since the surgery is on the right side. Long, good talk with my sister. I made her promise she would wake me up from the anesthesia, no matter what. She said not to worry, even if she has to fight with all of them, she will make sure I wake up. I feel so much support and love from her. I wish I could support her also in some way.

June 9—I can write! my hand is not immobilized!

The operation was yesterday. Before they took me to the operating room, I was shaking with fear. The anesthesia trip was weird; I was running wildly, out

---

[*] Later research proved that Dr. Clay was right!

of breath, and bumping against the walls of a long corridor. The walls were made of cork and every time I bumped against them there was a thump. At the end of the corridor there was freedom and health, and I was my healthy self, with no cancer and two breasts.

I hated the mask they put on my face. I felt like a big blob of protoplasm, abandoned in the recovery room for six hours. The nurses kept coming to check my blood pressure, but I felt unattended and unheard. I was tremendously thirsty and kept asking for water. Like a child I kept saying, "Please take me back to my room..."

Now I have an intravenous needle in the left arm and a drainage tube in my right side going from my chest to a machine in the wall. Today I should be able to walk a little. I have some pain in my chest and I took one painkiller. Last night there was a parade of people and telephone calls from many friends. I am reading *Sheila Levine is Dead and Living in New York*, and it made me laugh even in the middle of all this.

June 11—Sunday morning I made a big mistake. I glued Dr. Frazier to the armchair and bombarded him with a thousand questions. I ended more depressed than ever because I realized how little they know about the whole subject. It makes me shiver. My cancer is carcinoma of the ducts with highly differentiated cells, which is supposed to be in my favor. Sunday afternoon everybody came to visit and I got worried. When I see so many people worrying about me, it makes me think I am in a very difficult situation and that I need help. It makes me feel weak.

Yesterday, Dr. Frazier changed the bandages and I saw my mutilated chest for the first time. There is a long scar, stitched with a blue thread, like a fishing line and the chest looks flat, somewhat sunk. He looked at me while I was looking at my scar and afterward said, "you did fine. It is hard. . . ." There was another young doctor with him who followed the whole thing with blue and cold eyes. I hated him on the spot. I felt like I was a big scar, not a human being.

All the doctors are men and all the nurses are women. Only the doctors introduce themselves. The nurses just come out and do their work directly. I started to introduce myself to the nurses, but there are so many it is hard to keep track of all of them.

It is five days since the operation, and I still don't know the results of the lymph node biopsies. They say that even if one to three lymph nodes have been invaded by cancer, the prognosis is still good. My sister is amazed at the abundance and at the service at the hospital. The towels, the silverware, all stuff that we could rip off and take home. She said she now understands how some maids steal from their bosses, because they see lying around stuff that they would have to work hard to get money to buy. Amazing as it is, this is the first time she experiences this.

Later, Dr. Frazier came in saying, "I have not forgotten about you." Looking rather serious, he announced that six out of the eighteen lymph nodes were malignant. And he added, "But I am not going to slash my wrists over this." Shit. I will have to have radiation treatment. When Federico[*] called and asked about the test, I lied and said it was okay. No details. He started screaming, "Hurray, hurray!" on the phone. Today, again, too many visitors. Some of them seem really in bad shape. I almost feel like I

---

[*] My son Federico was 13 years old at the time.

have to reassure them that I am not dying yet. After everybody left, I cried a little. But I did it when I was sure I was going to be alone. I don't want the hospital staff to see me cry.

June 16—At home. When I came home, my eyes could not stand the brightness and the light in my house. I got myself to bed right away and when I woke up, it was dark. Next to the stitches under my axilla, there is a swollen piece of flesh. I worried for a while but when I showed it to my sister, she thought it looked like normal swelling and I got re-assured. I don't know what I would do without her.

June 17—Last night's dream made me very sad. I dreamed that my right breast had grown again, a lit-tle bit smaller, round like an adolescent's breast. As I touched it and marvelled, I was saying, "So they do grow again." Then somebody said, "No, they do not grow again." I was in the middle of a green field, trying to lift the corner of my desk, the desk of my teens. But I could not lift it, I could not lift the desk because my right arm was weak because of the scar. So the loss of the breast became real again.

June 20—Today I had my first shower since the oper-ation and my first real look at my body. Every time I look at myself in the mirror I get tears in my eyes; my body looks like a half-boy's body and a half-woman's body.

June 30—Things are moving really fast. My co-counselor came and I cried for a whole half-hour and the words I wanted to say were, "It's not my fault. I have not done anything wrong. I am not ashamed." I have been crying every day and feeling envious of people who do not have cancer. I said to her, "I wish you had cancer, too!" and then I cried even more thinking what a horrible person I must be to have said that to her. Luckily, she did not seem to mind.

My sister left yesterday. We almost managed to make her miss the plane. Her watch had stopped and we were at the Harvard Coop at 3:00 and her flight was leaving at 4:05. She made it!

July 1—Brigitte called. Fuck Brigitte. She wanted to tell me that big scars interfere with intimate relationships; she knows because her mother had a big scar and never again became physically intimate with anybody. And what about the lymph nodes? Do I have to wait five years before I know if I am cured? I put down the phone with rage. I decided she is an insensitive piece of wood—she just happens to look like a woman.

July 3—Yesterday was the worst since my operation. I went to this new clinic to start the radiation treatment. Dr. Hamilton was checking me out and she said that she would not have had a mastectomy. Then she realized that she had blown it and added that I was getting good treatment. She put me through a whole bunch of tests, x-rays of practically every part of my body, and set me up for a liver scan. Now I am really scared about what all these tests are going to show. I came home almost dead and then went out with Mary for supper. It turns out that the radiation treatment will be done at MIT! I hate MIT—it is so cold and patriarchal. And I get reminded of all the times that I went there to do experiments and felt inadequate and out of it.

July 4—Hot and muggy. It is after my first radiation treatment. They marked my chest with magic markers so that they know exactly which areas get the radiation. They strapped me into a chair, arms hanging from two support lifts and they fixed my head against a pole by wrapping a plastic strap around it. The chair swings back and forth in front of the radiation source. The room is dark and there are travel posters hanging on the walls; as the chair moves from one end of the room to the other, I go back and forth from Switzerland to London, Amsterdam, and Paris. They left me alone in the room and I felt like an astronaut in a space capsule.

I like the two women technicians. They tell us cancer stories with happy endings. The other patients are mostly middle-aged women and elderly men. We don't talk to each other. We go into the dressing rooms looking healthy and come out looking like patients, wearing our hospital gowns. The treatment takes fifteen minutes. But I resent having to come here and go through this. Somehow I feel cheated. They never talked about anything else but the mastectomy. Radiation only appeared in the picture after the lymph nodes were found to be malignant. To put it mildly, they did not prepare me for this shit.

July 7—Everybody is very surprised that the radiation treatment is not dragging me down and that I am doing so well. According to Dr. Hamilton, radiation should not have side effects. But, she added, "many housewives" find it very traumatic because they have to be there on time and they get emotionally hung up. And then she said, "But from the type of person you are and how you attack life," one would expect that I would not suffer from it. And so she set me up to be very different from those "housewives." She blew it again.

July 16—Another big mistake. I went to the dentist and he started screaming at me for not going to see him sooner, something about the bridge and how I brush my teeth. I felt like crying right in his office. I have to remember never again to see two doctors in the same day. I will just have to wait until I am done with radiation.

July 18—Liver scan. An intravenous injection of a radioactive isotope that gets followed by a gamma-ray detector and registered on a computer. A bit scary. While I was on the table lying down, the lymph nodes kept reappearing in my head and death statistics kept dancing in my eyes. I imagine lymph nodes looking like knots on a cord all tied up together. I hate to go to the hospital.

July 22—Liver scan was okay. I miss Federico. He has such good energy. It is harder to be going through this without him around. I want so much to live and to see him grow up and become a beautiful person. He still needs me, I cannot die yet.

1975

After the initial crisis of mastectomy and radiation, I started the long process of learning to live with the fear of recurrence. I went for check-ups, first every three months, then every six months. My internist was very optimistic about my situation and more than once stated that I was probably "cured." I went through periods of worrying incessantly about the cancer, but I also had periods when I was calm and believed that I was "through" with the whole experience.

April 20—This is a drag. After a whole year of co-counseling I am still crying about my breast. I am really tired about this whole thing. And what am I going to do this summer? I will have to get a special kind of bathing suit, or have something made for a regular one. What a bore.

November 27—After a check-up—all tests are normal and the mammography is fine, too. Hurrah! What else can I want?

1977

April—Three years from the mastectomy and every-thing is still okay. Could it be that I am really going to be well forever? They say that the first two years is the period when most recurrences appear, and that afterwards they are less common. But I do not trust the statistics.

September—Last weekend when I went camping on the Cape I had a coughing fit every time I lay down to sleep. I didn't feel like I had a cold. Maybe I am allergic to the goose down in the sleeping bag?

1978

April 27—Dr. Todd listened to my chest and ordered an x- ray. It was clean. Nothing to worry about. But my cough does not go away. I have been coughing since September and it does not get better. He shook his head and said to take some cough drops and asked me if I was tense and worried. Was something in my life bothering me? I said, yes, the cough was bothering me. He laughed and seemed unconcerned.

May 19—Dr. Todd sent me to see an allergist. They don't know what to do with me. The allergist says he won't treat me if I won't get rid of my cat. He suspects the cat is the origin of my cough. He is damned wrong. I have had Emma for five years with no problems. But he is fixed on it.

July 13—I spent the weekend in Nantucket with my friend Barbara, coughing and she finally noticed and said, "What's that all about?" I told her that I was going nuts with this cough and they keep saying it is nothing.

October 16—I saw this big specialist on respiratory diseases. He said I have a bad case of bronchitis and gave me a prescription. Well, we shall see, at least, this is some kind of diagnosis.

1979

January 13—My cough is so bad, I can't sleep. When I lay down it gets worse. I need two or three pillows to be able to stand it. I can't sleep more than two or three hours, and I also feel a lump in my left breast. I mentioned it to Nance, Dr. Todd's nurse practitioner, but she did not agree with me.

February 13—There is fluid in my lungs. They took it out and found cancer cells. Metastasis. I have metastatic breast cancer. My fight starts again. I suddenly feel very tired, and I just want to go to sleep and forget about all of this. They want to do an estrogen-receptor test on the liquid they took out of my lung. If the test is positive, they want to remove my ovaries. But if it is negative, they still want to remove my ovaries. So what is the purpose of the test? I can't get a straight answer. Somebody is confused, and I know it is not me. If the test is negative, it may simply be because there are not enough cancer cells, and I could still be estrogen-positive.[*]

February 17—Ann called and said that she recently met a woman at a co-counseling workshop who had metastatic liver cancer. Her uterus and lower part of the intestines were removed and she was given two months to live with chemotherapy. She refused chemo and did a lot of emotional discharge and went on the Kelly diet, and she has been well for the past six years. I called her up and indeed she confirmed the story. She gave me the name of the Kelly Foundation to write for information.

I made a list of 19 questions to ask the oncologist about the plan. He is not going to like it. And I am going to tell him that I want a consultant at the Sidney Farber Center with their experts on breast cancer. These specialists kill me. Sometimes I think I should look for a specialist on breast cancers of the right breast because if I get a specialist of the cancers of the left breast, it will be useless.

February 23—I finally got it that I have an incurable disease. Odd. I feel the same but now I am one of those with an incurable disease. It still does not make sense to me. Diane called and said that George in Philadelphia had cancer in the intestine, had chemo, and is now in remission and will talk to me if I wanted. I called him up and he was great. He said that he would go into the cancer treatment ward with his co-counselor and cry and shake dur-

---

[*] In 1974 when I had the mastectomy there was no ERT test available; that is why they did not know if my cancer is estrogen dependent or not.

ing the treatment. The other patients, all sitting quietly and obediently, were amazed. The nurses and doctors were in shock. He told me to read the Simonton book, *Getting Well Again,*[*] and create a support group. I started crying on the phone. I don't even know him, but I felt like I was talking to a member of my family, somebody really close and that he really cared about me. I hope I get to meet him sometime.

February 26—When I ask how long a remission I can get from removing my ovaries (if it works), I can't get a straight answer. One year two years, five years, ten. Anything goes. They just don't know. Case by case. I am on my own. But they all stress that it is a remission and not a cure, in case I had any illusions.

I went to the Quilapayun (a Chilean folklore music group) concert. It was dedicated to Victor Jara, the Chilean singer killed in the Santiago stadium during the coup against Allende. The spirit of the Chilean resistance lives! I went quite depressed, and by the end I was feeling much stronger.

March 2—I still feel a lump in my left breast and nobody seems to hear. The ERT test was negative, so I am going to have my ovaries removed not knowing if the tumor is sensitive to estrogen, after all. I just go and hope for the best. I told them that I don't want total anesthesia, I will have a spinal. They were very surprised, but I insisted, no more total anesthesia for me.

I went to see a nutritional consultant who does the Kelly diet. It is an expensive and elaborate affair:

---

[*] O. Carl Simonton, M.D., Stephanie Matthews-Simonton, and James Creighton, *Getting Well Again*, Los Angeles: J.P. Tarcher, 1978.

$200 initial investment, and then the costs for dietary supplements come $3,000–4,000 per year. Supplements every moment, before and after meals, in the middle of the night, etc. My old landlady and friend, Judith, sent me a friend of hers who is in a situation somewhat similar to mine. She came to visit and told me her story which was very moving. Four and a half years ago she was told she had six months to live; she was in her late thirties. She had everything done to her: bilateral mastectomy, oophorectomy, chemotherapy, Simonton work, you name it. A real fighter, another sister struggling for her life. I wish somebody would organize a big meeting of cancer patients; we could help each other a lot more if we were organized.

March 17—I am furious. After scheduling me for removal of the ovaries, I kept talking about my left breast, and finally at the last moment they want me to have a mammogram, and now I don't know what is going to happen. Am I going to have another mastectomy also? This is incredible. I am furious.

March 19—When Federico heard about the lump and the operation on the ovaries, he got mad at me. "Oh, mom, no! How can you take it?" I felt sad and could not say anything else.

In the hospital. Again, I have a private room, but the telephone is missing. Stolen, according to the nurse's assistant. The room looks like a room I had five years ago. I will leave this room. I will not die here.

March 23—After surgery. This time I was awake during the operation. Dr. Frazier sang Italian operas while cutting my body and tried to cheer me up with his energy. The lump is malignant. They keep asking me if I have hot flashes. I do. All of a sudden, from one day to the next, I have become menopausal.

April 1—My cough seems do be dimishing...

April 3—I sleep a lot. My cough is definitely better. I like the Simonton book. It gives me hope. There are, after all, things I can do to help myself. I am not a total victim.

April 9—The chest x-rays show some slight improvement (less fluid in the lungs), so it looks like the treatment is working. A modest and cautious hurrah. I went to Bread and Circus, the health food store, and the guy who works in the vitamin section told me his father has lung cancer and he has been "supplementing" him for a year, and he is doing very well. So I told him my story, and he told me what to get. It felt good to have somebody who does not know me try to help me, and it reminded me of when I was living in Europe. I had this friendly butcher who knew exactly what cuts of meat to give me.

Judy's friend called and said that two women are starting a group for women who have cancer. Do I want to go? I said yes. She says she does not have the energy to go. There are already three women interested.

May 18—The group was amazing. There is a woman with inoperable breast cancer, one with lung cancer, one with leukemia, and myself. The one with leukemia believes in mind control of the cancer, diet, the whole alternative approach, and has been well now for three years after almost dying. I like her a lot. She thinks she got herself well because she changed her lifestyle, abandoned a competitive career, an oppressive family and is now a feminist and a healer. Far out.

June 27—Last weekend I went to the Simontons' workshop. They brought their books alive for me. My head has been turned around. It seems that I can do a lot to get myself well. I don't have anything to lose. I will try their approach. At their workshop I picked up a leaflet put out by two women. They have formed a local group called Cancer Counseling Associates, and they do counseling to cancer patients, groups for patients, family and friends, and training in stress reduction: relaxation techniques, meditation, active imagination, and goal setting. One of the two women, Ann, had metastatic breast cancer herself and has now been well for three years with no evidence of disease. She interests me. I want to work with someone who knows how it feels to have cancer. How people treat you differently and how lonely it feels. They have both trained with the Simontons in Texas, and the one with cancer has worked with them as a co-leader. I am going to check her out. I have been doing the relaxations and visualizations on my own, but sometimes I feel lost and don't know if I am on the right track. I can surely use some help.

When I imagine who is helping me fight the cancer, images of my women friends appear. The only men who have come to help me are Fidel Castro and Che Guevara! I just finished reading Che Guevara's *Reminiscences of the Cuban Revolutionary War*, and I felt that we were both fighting for our lives. He is in the Sierra Maestra, and me at home. I paid attention to his strategy, how he kept his morale high, how he persisted, how he would not accept defeat. I felt accompanied. I felt I am not alone.

August 3—I have been seeing Ann for a few weeks for individual therapy and for suggestions on how to use the Simontons' ideas. I got very angry in my first session and she thought that was great, that all that energy is going to help me fight the cancer. I have been reading Rose Kushner's* book about breast cancer and realized that five years ago when they did my mastectomy they did not "stage" me. They did the operation and only afterward checked about cancer spread. That was wrong because if the cancer had spread already, the mastectomy would have been totally unnecessary. Luckily, there was no spread then, but still, it shows that they were not thinking well. And, moreover, now I know that the mastectomy and radiation did not cure me, so I may be in worse shape now because of those 21 radiation treatments.

Becoming aware of my mortality has been a sobering experience. I don't think I faced it so clearly five years ago, when I still thought I may be cured. And then the discovery that life is terminal for everybody, not just for me. Physical death is going to happen to everybody alive, and every single human being will have to face her or his death. So we are all in the same boat, though it looks like I have become "mortal," while everybody else is still "immortal."

August 20—The cough keeps getting better, and in the last chest x-rays they did not see any more fluid in my lungs. The treatment is working.

What I like about this Simonton thing is that it gives me an active role to play. Doctors, hospitals, the whole scenario is so disempowering that it stimu-

---

* Kushner, Rose, *Why Me? Breast Cancer: A Personal History and an Investigative Report* (New York: Harcourt Brace Jovanovich, 1975).

lates all my victim feelings. They even call us "cancer victims..." But the idea that one can contribute to one's own health, even in the case of cancer, that one can mobilize all of one's resources, is an exciting one. Just thinking about it makes me feel stronger and less afraid. So, I have started changing the way I eat. I threw away all my aluminum cookware and got iron or steel. I threw away sugar, coffee, and all cans and preserved food. A good diet has to help my body, though the Simontons don't talk about diet, and I suspect they are into junk food themselves. To increase my body's healing ability and to learn how to relax and have more fun seem like nice goals for me!

What I don't like about the Simonton model is the possibility of "blaming the victim"—that is, of saying that I brought the cancer on myself because I did not live right. And sometimes it feels that way. That it was my psychological make-up that made me vulnerable. I don't like that feeling, and I don't think it is right. There is all this stuff about how nice people get cancer. The idea is that being nice prevents you from expressing anger or other negative emotions, and that brings the cancer on. Too simplistic, though. But sometimes I feel that is what Ann is saying, or better, she does not say it, but she implies it.

December 3—Cough is almost completely gone, just a little bit when I lay down. And I feel pretty good. I have been training myself to do physical exercise at least three times a week, for at least an hour and I keep up my relaxation-visualizations about three times a day.

December 7—Today I got scared again. I had a bad coughing fit, like I used to have months ago, but it came all of a sudden and it may be that I am getting a cold. After all, I have to remind myself that I can get other illnesses.

December 9—I decided to treat myself to a massage. I felt very shy when I made the appointment. I thought I should tell the woman before I went that I had only one breast so that she would not be shocked or scared. But I could not find the words over the phone. So I just went, and before taking my clothes off I said to her, "I have only one breast because I have cancer, and my ovaries were taken away also." She did not blink an eye and afterward told me that she has seen all kinds of bodies in all kinds of shapes, and I felt accepted and just like one more regular person. But it was scary beforehand. I liked her a lot.

1980

January 3—I had a terrible dream. In the dream, Federico had cancer. It had shown in some x-rays. I started to cry in the middle of the street in total despair, saying, "My son, my only son, look what happened to him!" And then Polly, one of his teachers in high school, came over and said that it was not so bad. No big deal. That the kind of cancer he had was made too much of, but in reality it was not so bad. She made it look like there was not going to be any problem, nothing to worry about.

January 6—Ann wants to start a health group for women. So instead of seeing her individually, I would be in a group with two other women, one who has leukemia and another one who has an uncommon thyroid disease, not life-threatening but potentially serious. I felt bad about the idea of ending my individual therapy, but Ann needs to do this because of her work at school (she is going to social work school), and she needs the time. I said that I might want once in a while, an individual session and she agreed. We'll see how this goes.

February 3—The group has been meeting at each one of our houses. Hearing the other women's horror stories makes me feel less lonely, and I also think that it might be useful because I will have to deal with other people and not just with Ann. The two women are friendly, and there is potential here, I think.

February 15—I have been feeling the group was not working so well for me. Elizabeth and Judy talk a lot, and a couple of times I found myself at the end of the session with very little time for myself. I was being polite, but I resented it. I felt that Ann was not watching and keeping track of the time, so in the next session I brought it out as a complaint. I said that I did not feel I was being paid enough attention, and I blamed her for not standing for my rights. Her answer was strong and right on. She pointed out to me that is exactly what I have to learn in a group— how to take care of my own needs, to speak up and not to let myself be run over. She is there to help us understand what is going on, and what is going on here is that I did not take responsibility for myself and I am blaming her. She is not my mother, and I am not a baby. I will never forget this answer. I will never again let myself not speak up. Even if I only remember this piece, I think the group has been worthwhile. I feel like I got something that could only be learned by going through the process that I went through. I know I will not forget this lesson easily.

May 7—I do not like the way that Ann looks. She has a grayish color in her face, and sometimes she has pain in her back on the sides of her spine. She does not go back for check-ups; she stopped seeing medical people three years ago and has never gone back. I feel uncomfortable because I am afraid she might be sick again and not be facing it. She does not want to hear about going for a consultation, and I think she looks really sick. What is going on here?

June 1—I am real worried about Ann. She looked terrible at our last meeting. The color on her face was death-like. I am simply not satisfied with the explanation she gave us about her condition. For me, she has not ruled out that it is cancer again. I called the other women in the group to tell them about how I feel, but Judy did not even want to hear about it. If I have learned one thing from Ann, it is this: to stick to my guns, to listen to what I really think. And this inner voice is now telling me that there is something not totally clear here.

June 25—Fred (Ann's husband) called last night. Ann is in the hospital. She has tumors in her spine. She was hospitalized in emergency last Saturday; her vital organs are not affected. They are trying to save her spine. I was not surprised. I fervently hoped that it would not be cancer, but somehow I knew.

June 30—I went to see Ann at the hospital. She looked very pale and unfriendly. I called before I went to make sure she wanted to see me. She asked why I had come, and I told her the truth—that I like her, support her, and thought maybe she would like to see me. She said she did want to see me and that I was the only person she had combed her hair for. She also said that she found it very uncomfortable to see me. She wanted to know what I thought of "the whole thing" and what I was doing for fun. I felt she was still trying to be my therapist and expected me to do all the talking, that she was not giving anything of herself. When I said I was leaving, she said "Good," and seemed relieved. And then she warned me not to work too hard, to enjoy myself. On the table, next to the bed, was a picture of her and her husband, looking young and happy. She treated the nurse with hostility and was clearly into being a pest. I hope it helps. I think this will be the last time I will see her.

July 3—I am very sad and worried about Ann. She is probably dying. My role model, my teacher for the last year. I learned so much from her. She had been working on a manuscript about her story, her recovery from cancer, and she was having trouble finishing it. I now know why. She probably knew her story was not finished, that the pain she was having was serious. In spite of her denial to us, she knew.

September 12—Helen, the therapist I met in Texas, and I have been talking about giving a three-month course for women who want to work on their health, using the Simonton ideas and incorporating a feminist perspective. We have collected articles, prepared a reading list, and designed a leaflet. We will do it at the feminist therapy collective which she is part of. I think my experience in co-counseling and my dealing with my cancer will give me enough strength to do this work. I am interested in seeing if this approach is helpful to other women, and I want to learn more about how to facilitate empowerment. But I will have to watch out that I don't get into helping others at the expense of myself. A delicate balance.

October 3—Yesterday we started the group. Eight women with different kinds of health problems. It is exciting for me to be doing this. To test these ideas in a feminist setting. The women seem very open to acknowledging the importance of one's emotional life in connection with physical health. And they are eager to learn better ways of handling one's life.

November 20—I hope I can convey to the group what has been the most important learning I have done in connection with my cancer. For me, through the illness experience, there has been a shift in the center of power and decision-making that affects and extends to all areas of my life. I consult with the medical profession and other "experts," but frankly I see myself as the final source of authority and decision-making regarding my illness. I believe that the views that the doctors have about cancer, their own fears and their sense of frustration can play a role in the course of the disease. And so I protect myself from their emotional hang-ups. I believe that in my case, as a result of accepting that mind, body, and spirit are one, my life has been enriched. Having to take charge of my life around the cancer has made me stronger and has certainly clarified my priorities. The cancer is not the greatest problem in my life. It is one serious problem, but it is just one more arena in which I have to play my life. This is an incredible feeling, but it is truly how I feel. What makes it hard is that in the eyes of the rest of the world, I am a cancer victim and people either get turned off or worry or get scared. That is why it is tempting to "pass" and say nothing about my cancer. "Passing" is a way to avoid having to deal with other people's fears and projections. Sometimes I feel like an actress who knows the whole play while the others are not aware yet of what their parts are in the drama.

1984: Conclusion

January—Ann died in January of 1981. My cough has almost completely disappeared, though sometimes I still have coughing spells. I am technically "in remission" with my cancer, a state that can end at any moment if a new recurrence is found. I have continued to improve the quality of my life, being kind to myself, and most importantly, being true to my feelings and wishes. Regarding the medical establishment, I left Dr. Todd for another doctor, an oncologist who seems more receptive to my reports about what I feel is going on with my body. I go for check-ups and I keep learning from the cancer.

Ann's death was a sobering reminder that no single approach can ensure the continuation of one's health—that we have, after all, a limited amount of power over the physical aspects of illness. What I learned from her was invaluable. She gave me support, intelligent criticism, and encouragement to stand for myself and to trust my intuition and my strength.

Facing the life-and-death struggle that cancer is has made the past ten years the most intense years of my life. I have never felt so alone and at the same time, so strong. Now when I get depressed or scared about my cancer coming back, I take a deep breath, try to relax, and remind myself to live "one day at a time." Which is, after all, all that any of us can count on.

Air Born

Portia Cornell

Arden often forgot over the summer just how awful her asthma attacks could be. When the weather was warm, she never wheezed. It was the chill of winter that got into her lungs and hung on with a death grip. And then there was her sister's breast cancer that suddenly appeared in July that threw them both into a tizzy.

After Vicky's mastectomy, Arden did what any sister would do: took her for chemotherapy shots, read up on the latest health theories on cancer, made an appointment with a naturopath, and bought some relaxation/visualization tapes. She shopped for dark green and yellow vegetables and changed to a diet of eating fish. August afternoons, they lay on the living room rug relaxing to healing tapes. Listening to soft music, imagining safe places to go, seeing white light surrounding their bodies. It had the soothing effect, they remarked, of being in church, although neither of the unmarried sisters had been to church in years. With this first threat to life and love she had ever really experienced, it was no wonder Arden forgot to renew her asthma inhaler prescription before the cold weather set in.

The elderly sisters had lived together for twenty years and they grew very close that summer. One morning Arden got out the big cardboard box of family photographs and found the one of them in rompers looking just like twins even though Vicky was two years younger. And there was that picture of their parents glowering at each other in front of the Christmas tree.

"I never felt they loved each other," said Vicky.

"They didn't raise us. We raised each other," said Arden.

"Remember when you went to the joke store and bought fake doggy-doo and left it on Mom's bed. When we heard her scream, we ran into our bedroom giggling," said Vicky. They laughed all through dinner over that one.

One cool October evening, Arden went outside to gather a few well-seasoned apple logs from the woodpile. The blue jays careened wildly through the last of the shriveling oak leaves. Arden carried the wood cradled in her arms.

"Don't forget to open the damper," warned Vicky as Arden lay the logs upon the grate. Arden felt a stiffness up the side of her neck. She wished Vicky wouldn't tell her what to do. It was bad enough to be doing all the housework now. Vicky always had to put in her two cents worth. She was sick and tired of it.

"How's Victoria feeling?" the teller asked in a hushed voice at the bank.

"How's your sister?" inquired the check out clerk at the supermarket.

It was tiresome taking care of a sick person, tiresome putting up a caring front, tiresome running all the errands. Most of all it was tiresome holding in the grief, like a toxic cloud, the fear that she might lose her sister, that she was helpless against the whim of illness and the punishment of loss.

Arden shoved ragged scraps of kindling under the logs and jabbed clumps of paper in between. She struck a match, fascinated by the hungry orange flames licking at the wood. Turning, she saw Vicky asleep on the couch, her gray curls clustered about her flushed cheeks. She looked dear and sweet as her baby photos.

"Vicky finds it hard not participating in our regular routine," Arden thought. "She says things because she feels left out. I should try to be nicer to her, poor thing."

She crept into the big crewel work wing chair and sat with her legs tucked under her navy gabardine skirt watching the tones on the walls blend from gray to blue as darkness slipped in and the sweet smell of applewood smoke curled into the night.

At her first cough, Arden knew she was reacting allergically to the smoke. It was as if the shadows in the room were blocking air from her lungs. When she tried to breathe air out, it sounded like the high-pitched whine of a baby in a far-off crib. She knew there was no pharmacy open to get the inhalers to clear her lungs. She huddled in the darkened room, her chest heaving, and she panicked. She remembered waking last night, panting, believing there was a dark figure standing at the foot of her bed. She had been dreaming, but the fear wouldn't go away.

At the allergist's office they had advised her in case of an attack: Get warm, relax, and breathe into your diaphragm. Arden rose and scraped the screen across the fire. Vicky didn't stir. She quietly closed the door to her bedroom, and lay down on her bed still wheezing.

She thought back to what her doctor said caused asthma. "It's an allergy you've developed, mostly genetic," he said.

But she knew from her reading that it was partially psychological. "Suppressed rage and grief," the books said.

Once her father grabbed her at the swimming pool when she was four to teach her to swim. She pulled away. She didn't trust him to hold her up. He promised he wouldn't let go of her in the water. But he did. She sputtered and choked until he pulled her out. She was furious. Her mother called her stubborn and she knew why. She didn't trust her parents would take care of her.

"I felt so alone as a child," Vicky had told her just that morning. "I was so glad I had you." They hugged each other.

Arden spoke with her allergist about nonmedical asthma remedies, like vitamin B_6 and E and herbs like coltsfoot and mullein. He sighed and said, "My dear, you think too much. Just go home and relax."

She did. Immediately. Slamming the door. Arden was as stubborn with him as she had been with her parents.

Lying in the dark, she made a bargain. If she overcame her asthma, Vicky could stop her cancer. It was all a matter of attitude. She believed she would not die from an attack. She thought of it as a trial initiation. She would decode the secrets of her symptoms and free herself, and Vicky as well.

Arden raised the window, sucking in night air. The moon, almost full, had turned the yard into a tangle of branches. Through the sodden air, pending with rain, came the coo of a mourning dove somewhere above.

There was a tap at Arden's door. "Are you in there?" It was Vicky.

Arden stiffened. "Just having a little asthma from the fire," she called. "I'm O.K."

But she knew she wasn't. Knew if she made it through that night without having to go to the hospital for a shot of epinephrine she was lucky. Release from this terror of drowning in air would come, if she relaxed and fell asleep, but with this continual gasping that was impossible. She felt she was fighting something: maybe her parents, maybe her allergist, maybe her own rage.

Adjusting her headphones, she slipped a relaxation tape into her cassette recorder. Soft music flowed in, then a voice: "Relax your toes, relax your calves. . ." Arden could feel herself beginning to relax. Then the tape ended, her breath quickened and the fear returned. She clicked in another tape, this time a visualization of the beach. She heard the swish of surf, pictured an immense blue apron of ocean, took comfort in the mewing of gulls.

She wondered if her asthma was created by a distrust of the air she was born into. She groaned and rolled over face down. In desperation she tried prayer: "Our Father who art in heaven, hallowed be thy name . . ." She was surprised she recalled it. "Thy will be done . . ." She actually felt a little loosening of her tight breath, so she repeated, "Thy will be done . . ."

Clicking on the tiny white lamp, she pulled some Buddhist meditations out from a pile of bedside books and opened it.

She read, "Feel the place of anger in your heart. How it hardens." She could feel that hardness. Her chest felt like it was covered with armor.

She read on, "Visualize someone for whom you hold anger." Vicky came to mind. She felt surprised and guilty. She would rather die than be angry at her sick sister.

She kept reading, "Now picture someone for whom you have great love." Again she was surprised, for this time she saw her high school drama teacher standing in a faded blue blouse and brown skirt, reciting lines from Shakespeare:

"The quality of mercy is not strained. It droppeth as the gentle rain from heaven upon the place beneath; It is twice blest; It blesseth him that gives and him that takes . . ." Arden sighed. Those were

some of her favorite lines in literature. Was she asking for mercy? she wondered.

She read on: "Extend this love to someone with
whom you have problems." Arden remembered feeling angry at Vicky—or was it the cancer that had
invaded here sister's body? That was it, she was
angry at Vicky because she was afraid she would
leave her all alone. She felt a rush of love for Vicky.

The meditation said, "Hold this person within
your heart." As Arden did this, she saw her mother
and father there with her sister holding her hand on
each side. Arden felt herself breaking, giving in, letting go.

"Extend this love to yourself, using your name."
Arden did so, whispering. And then she saw them
all together, her mother who called her stubborn, her
father whom she never trusted, her sister who threatened to leave her and herself full of her usual rage.

"The quality of mercy is not strained," thought
Arden. Tears dropped gently down upon her cheeks.
"And I am twice blessed because I can take as well
as give." She breathed deeply. Her shoulders
drooped and her eyelids fluttered down like gulls
settling on the shore of an immense blue apron.

Later Vicky tiptoed into Arden's room and saw
her bathed in the white light of the lamp, asleep
with an open book in her hand. She seemed to be
smiling. She was dreaming of herself as a new born
baby gurgling at life. Vicky crossed the room and
closed the window. The rain had begun.

Live and Let Live

Laura Post

I saw her today. No matter how often I have visited her, I still cannot get used to the noises or to having slow, written conversations with her because she is still breathing with a machine and cannot speak.

I am a doctor; I have spent many hours in the Intensive Care Unit, yet I remain uncomfortable with Celine. But let me begin at the beginning.[*]

▲ ▲ ▲

I was two months short of sixteen when my father died of lung cancer. In fact, he didn't even die of the lung cancer per se, but of the brain metastases. Well, actually, he didn't die of the cancer at all—directly, anyway—he killed himself. But that is another story.

Fifteen years later, I am armed with medical jargon, buffered by the multitude of cancer sicknesses and other deaths I have witnessed during my five years of medical school and internship. With three more years of training as a psychiatrist, I have learned about all the possible defenses to being confronted with the ultimate form of loss. Many of the intervening, unaccounted-for years I spent burying my own feelings in work and drink. Maybe this is why Celine's illness hit me so hard: saying goodbye to her is my first sober experience of human passing.

---

[*] Dramatic liberties have been taken with this true story and changes have been made to protect the patient's identity.

Copyright © 1991 by Laura Post

▲ ▲ ▲

Several days later Celine was groggy from pain medications and able to write only a few words. I felt disappointment at her not being able to respond—an old sadness, an aloneness with urgent emotions that I may have to deal with on my own.

Celine's ventilator was to be disconnected soon, and I felt somewhat responsible for this fate. But let me really start at the beginning.

▲ ▲ ▲

I met Celine more than a year ago. Born in China to a Japanese mother and Chinese father, raised in the cloistered sanctuary of the French religious, Celine remained skeptical of many Western approaches to her chronic and worsening back pain. Her reliance on many healers—Chinese, American, Vietnamese—had persisted as long as I had known her. Her many mistrusts permeated our discussions about her lost music,* her fractured ties with her "sadly Americanized" sister, and her forced lapse with her beloved uncle, a former, high-ranking government official detained until July 1990 in the aftermath of the Vietnam conflict. Celine and I spoke of many things. I felt her loneliness—treated as a stranger in a strange land, she was a stranger to herself—her dis-ease with mainstream, Western society and its misogynistic, xenophobic, racist beliefs. My own—a white American lesbian psychiatrist's—oppression-consciousness was sharpened through her.

Much of Celine's pain was expressed through her body—for reasons that were cultural, personal, and physiological. After she had complained about her

---

* She had been an opera singer in the 1960s and 70s.

persistent low back pain, I suggested that she seek out a neurosurgeon. Her internist had given her a clean bill of health after routine blood tests. The neurosurgeon whom Celine eventually approached discovered a mass in Celine's lower spine which turned out to be a metastasis of a malignant cancer. Celine began to speak often of her wish to see her uncle once more.

An exhaustive series of invasive and painful diagnostic procedures failed to uncover the source of the cancer, thus increasing Celine's psychic pain—fear about the unknown. What was known, statistically anyway, was that Celine had, perhaps, a five-percent chance of living more than six months. Because of her accent and 'foreign' culture, Celine's medical doctors were unsure that Celine comprehended their messages about treatment variables and possibilities.

As someone who knew Celine well, I was recruited to help decide whether to disconnect Celine from her respirator (after which her medical doctors predicted that she would die within a few days). Another possibility was aggressive, difficult, possibly painful rehabilitation in a nursing home after a new surgery to place a permanent breathing tube in her throat,* replacing the temporary breathing tube in her mouth.

I have worked in the hospice setting; I have worked with very ill people with AIDS. I have used the words "peace and dignity" with patients who wanted, in the nurturing glow of their loved ones, to let go and move on. I knew that, in Celine's case, her surgeons did not believe that her uncle would ever come from Vietnam, had no faith in her ability to struggle and recover, perceived no meaning in her quiet life. The peace and dignity that I saw had

---

* This procedure is called a tracheostomy.

much to do with causing no more suffering from her cancer pain but also had to do with choosing a path untainted by pain from the ignorance and insensitivity of her medical doctors.

Celine's nephew told me his understanding of Celine's wish to not suffer any more on earth. Pages of notes that Celine had written to me while she was in the hospital asked for no more surgery, and no more pain, though she still yearned for life and home. When first asked to help Celine, I spoke with Celine, with her nephew, with the ICU nurses; I reread my medical texts, I talked with several oncologists.

When after days of deliberation and re-discussion, Celine asked me what I really thought, I told her that I respected her and her wishes and made sure that she understood why the temporary breathing tube in her mouth couldn't remain and why another surgery and then rehabilitation were being considered. I tried to translate into her sense of pain what another surgery and breathing tube care would cost her and what it might be like for her to be in a nursing home. I told her that, if she chose surgery, rehab, and nursing home, it might not be as bad as she imagined but that I didn't want to direct her, only to inform and affirm. I told her that I thought that the surgery for the permanent breathing tube was less than what she had already endured, that she could tolerate another surgery and rehabilitation, but that I did not know what was best. I told her that I would support her decision to accept or to forego further treatment, and I promised that I would continue to visit her regardless of her choice, and help her remaining time and ultimate death be peaceful and dignified. Celine decided that she wanted to go ahead with the surgery and rehab, even with the nursing home, as long as I would support her. She believed that seeing her uncle once more would bring her peace and dignity; she had faith that I could arrange everything.[*]

Celine's surgical team had told her that she had endured a lot and that further surgery and rehab would cause her pain. They believed that Celine was using valuable resources that could be "more appropriately applied." I told the team of Celine's most sacred dream, of seeing her uncle once more before she died. Nevertheless, their intention, regardless of Celine's wishes or mine, was to do no tracheostomy and to disconnect the respirator. Their actions would kill Celine; I wanted her to feel some control over her death.

What I said then to Celine was not a spontaneous reply to her queries but a carefully-worded opinion for a definite purpose. I used her great trust in me to lead her to a choice about the timing and manner of her death. When, worn down by the surgeons, Celine again asked my views, I reported that her medical doctors told me that she probably would not be able to tolerate the pain or even live as long as six more months even with the surgery and rehab and that six months might not be enough time to arrange for her newly-liberated uncle in Vietnam to come to the U.S. I told her that she could choose to have no more surgery, no permanent breathing tube, no painful rehabilitation, that such a choice was what her nephew and her doctors told me they thought best. I knew, but did not say, that the ICU doctors harbored the most definite intention of disconnecting the ventilator several days later. Celine changed her mind and decided that she wanted to disconnect the respirator.

---

[*]   I was Celine's therapist.

Celine seemed to accept her new fate, gave up on seeing her uncle, and offered a new last wish: to be able to talk with me. What she wanted was for the respirator to be disconnected, in my presence, and to be able to speak, not write, with me before she died, in peace and dignity.

She did not get that wish, either. After that difficult visit, I never saw her again. Her doctors disconnected the ventilator very soon thereafter, without contacting me.

▲ ▲ ▲

Celine is dead, not by suicide or any of the other self-destructive actions that most commonly claim the lives of therapists' patients. She died naturally, without artificial life support; she made her own decision about when to die. I hope that she died with her nephew close by. I had wished to be there for the final goodbye, but they did not call me when the respirator was disconnected.

As I write, I know that she gave me her permission to pass on her story. This is my story too. I remember her voice, the progress of our work together, her tangible gifts to me: last Thanksgiving, she sang me a song she had written about a beautiful woman. The image of her humming to the nurses (all female) when they bathed and cared for her; the nurses' whispers to me that she was "psychologically OK"; that they thought that she could tolerate one more small surgery to be able to speak goodbyes.

I am a physician. I am a psychiatrist. I have been through this process of dying with somebody I love before. I understand the financial, medical, and psychological issues; I know where to go for answers, for support. Yet the effective power within the medical establishment is not mine.

After that last visit, one of Celine's medical doctors took me aside. I wanted consolation for my loss, empathy for my difficult decisions, affirmation for my continued good work with Celine. Instead, he lauded my helpfulness in continuing to visit Celine "even though she was dying"—and apparently in his opinion no longer my patient or even someone to whom I would continue to feel connected. He praised my assistance in helping the team come to a "satisfactory resolution" and asked the name of my supervisor so that he could make a favorable report about me.*

The difficulty in this situation was not about gender-biased hierarchy, at least not only about that. The two most helpful doctors on Celine's treatment team, one male and one female, were interns, without enough power to make a difference and not sufficiently advanced in their training to have lost all their feelings about their patients. The young male doctor was tearful and quavery-voiced in talking with me about Celine; the young female doctor, perhaps as a way of pushing aside her own troubling emotions, took on many tasks to help reconnect Celine and her friends. But neither of those doctors called to let me know what was happening over the weekend with Celine or even to let me know that she had died. One less patient, next case.

The real issue, to me, is emotional clarity. Encouraging other doctors to allow their feelings to come and to be a part of their decisions. To be present with other people, to connect around real issues beyond academic discussions of the tragedy of can-

---

* He did make such a report.

cer, statistics, and differing cultural responses to radiation and chemotherapy. I cried in feeling close to
Celine; I was saddened by her illness yet pleased at
her decision to struggle on with me. I was able to
hold that feeling and to my own hopes only briefly
before they succumbed to the familiar, intellectual
insistence of my medical peers, before I allowed Celine to act out their wishes and give up.

I have lost Celine. I have lost my self, temporarily,
in one more battle with the rational. I cry now at
many losses that I think I could have made easier, at
what I wish I had done, not done, or done differently. I reclaim Celine in my story as I become
stronger in my determination to honor my own
truth despite odds, anger, rejection. I do not know
whether Celine would have lived through what was
ahead; I know that I will live and feel and thrive.

▲ ▲ ▲

I had thought that this story was finished. My
grandmother told me today that she has cancer.

Legacy[*]

Nicky Morris

When I was eight my mother felt a lump in her
breast the size of a small pea, saw a doctor, checked
herself into a private hospital room because no public beds were available, had a radical mastectomy,
and put me and my brother in an orphanage. I went
to visit her in the hospital, and my memory is that
everything was gray. The only color I remember for
years of my childhood is the color of the grounds of
her convalescent home—bright greens, flowers, and
the sun shedding yellow over everything.

For weeks I have put off writing about my
mother's cancer and the effect it had on me because
I was afraid everything I'd say would come out dry,
uninteresting, much like I experienced my childhood. Just the barest facts. Now I feel for the child
who was alone too young, and too terrified to feel
anything but the world as a gray, bare place. There
was no one to take us in when my mother was sick,
would have been no one if she had died, which she
expected to.

She never told me she had cancer but by the time
she mentioned it, almost in passing, I had deduced
it. I didn't know until a few months ago that when I
was a child she had expected to die, that the breast
cancer had metastasized and was in her lymphatic
system. When she told me it made sense of my experience in the orphanage where I was afraid to go to
sleep, and in the boarding school I was sent to after

---

[*] This article originally appeared in *Sojourner*.

143

the orphanage where, longing for her, I cried all the time, dreamed often that she had died, and was terrified that I was going to be left alone in the world, and that the world was ending. She hoped that I would find a home at the boarding school and that I would learn to be independent. And I suppose I did learn after a fashion, looking for a boy to want me, and, after the first term, making pacts with myself over how long I could go without crying. It was not a happy place, and when I was sixteen I ran away to get married.

Sometimes I wonder if things would have been different for me if my mother had told me that she had cancer and that she thought she was dying. Perhaps they would have. The quality of hidden secrets that pervaded my childhood was difficult, but what sense could I have made of a dying mother?

When I was in my early twenties, doctors started telling me I had a very high risk of cancer because my grandmother had died of premenopausal breast cancer and because my mother was supposed to have died of it. One doctor recommended preventative mastectomies of both breasts. I began to be terrified I was going to get it, lose my breasts, perhaps even die. I'd dream I was in a cancer ward, and during the day I would catch myself fantasizing about being in hospital, dying. What I would do, where I would find pain-killing drugs, would my lover stay with me, how would my daughter manage: these were questions I would ask myself all the time. I tried to eat less fat and was ashamed to examine my breasts. Ashamed and afraid. Then I would feel guilty about even thinking about having cancer because so many women actually do have it. What right do I have to be imagining I am dying?

My mother says that having cancer was the best thing that ever happened to her. I believe her, although I don't quite understand. I do know that now she is doing what she wants to do with her life. She has moved home to the village where she grew up, and is painting and designing. The cancer was certainly not the best thing that ever happened to me. My legacy is that to some extent I believe that I carry the cancer within me, waiting to get me. I don't live my life fully; I am tentative and afraid often. I want to be free.

What happened to me was because of a terrible disease, one that my mother believes is caused by stress, in her case the stress of being a single parent with no family to support her in a society that despised women alone with children. But what happened to me was also because of that same society, one not organized to provide the care that the children of cancer patients need to flourish. I am sure there are many people like me, children who grew up unnecessarily afraid and alone.

Now when I hear of a woman with cancer I tell her about my mother, how she survived so fully that the doctors say that if she has cancer now it is a new disease. The woman who was supposed to die and didn't. Her presence gives hope, but the cost was still enormous.

Real Life?

Wendy Ann Ryden

Because forgetfulness has too high a price in the end—that is why I write this, because I cannot write anything else.

The dual life I have been living—the schism between family and friends; desires and obligations; writer and daughter; adult and child—has reached its apex. I have become two people, as distinct as people can be, in the same body.

One person is the woman in her apartment who lives normally—applies for jobs, meets deadlines, reads books, watches baseball, has sex—who lives as most of us usually live, with a feeling of perpetualness, characters in a book. She lives without death.

The other is the daughter who goes home to watch her mother die of cancer. It took some time for these separate and distinct personalities to emerge. One week I think it took.

One week after the prognosis of six months was given. Perhaps if I hadn't convinced myself that the mastectomy would be the worst of it, then, perhaps it would have taken even less time. Shock. Incredulity. Numbness. Multiple personalities emerge as a manifestation of denial—one of the psyche's defense mechanisms which protect us from disparate images we have of ourselves in relation to reality. Any psychology textbook will tell you this strategy is clearly an unacceptable one.

But we don't always have control.

There is no order to this story. I warn you from the start, there is no order to what has happened. A

147

chronology could be imposed, certainly, served up, dished out, swallowed…but there is no order.

▲ ▲ ▲

My mother's stomach is enormous, enormous as a pregnant woman's belly, a pregnant woman who is too fat, fatter than her doctor would have liked. Such a woman would have trouble returning to her pre-pregnant state (she would probably have been warned of this catastrophe), but if she breast-feeds, her chances of breast cancer lessen. That doesn't always work, though. Four children, my mother had four breast-fed children. I don't plan to have any. No protection. High-risk group. I will definitely get it. My stomach will become as bloated and pregnant-looking, as swollen with tumor as my mother's is now, despite my attempts to organize my life so that that would never happen.

▲ ▲ ▲

This is the daughter. The daughter pushes the bed-pan under her mother. (They say the mother should be able to live the next few months if she has a good attitude, if she wants to live, if she has something she wants to live for. There is no reason she cannot get out of bed. My mother has a terrible attitude: she will not get out of bed, she will not be cheerful and brave and fight to live. She prays to God that she will die soon.) The mother's legs are bent up like she is on the examining table, feet in stirrups, legs spread. She has almost no pubic hair left. Do we lose our pubic hair as we get older, the daughter wonders. Is it the disease? The daughter's genital hair is dark and oily and thick and grows down the inside of her thighs. Her sister's is light brown, not so thick, is contained to the pubic region. Does it turn gray, pubic hair, when we get older? The mother is 62 and has very few gray hairs on her head. The mother has always looked younger, the daughter has always counted on the mother living for a long, long time, just shy of forever.

The mother has no shame. She is in too much pain and too much despair to have shame. She lies in her bed, wearing nothing but a short robe she lets hang wide open. With a sheet we cover what she exposes.

The mother cries.

The daughter cries as the mother cries as the father cries and whoever else is visiting that day.

Then the daughter leaves because Eros beats out Thanatos, instinct for self-preservation takes over. While she is driving the car, the other personality begins to emerge and take responsibility for the organism.

▲ ▲ ▲

I go to teach the summer night class I have been teaching for the past few weeks. Hearing the death sentence was the same as hearing a death announcement, and I was unable to go to class that particular evening. Still, I was concerned about propriety; I wanted to do the right thing. My friend called the school office for me, but, as I found out later, no one bothered to notify my class that I was not coming. Well, I have never liked this place. I make a decision: I won't teach here anymore; I'll look for a new job. When this is all over…

Fortunately I don't have much more work left to prepare for this course, so I am not jealous of the time I devote to her. In the first few days, before the split, nothing interfered with my concern for my mother. I went to the hospital every day and stayed with her from noon to six o'clock. I would have stayed the extra two hours allowed visitors, except my sister would persuade me to leave for dinner.

She was not so sick then, immediately following the operation.

She was still my mother then.

I was still one person.

The tumor in the liver had not yet expanded her stomach, her ankles had not yet puffed up to twice their size, the whites of her eyes were not quite so yellow.

Immediately following the operation she didn't yet know she would never get better. No one actually told her. The doctor didn't want to because of her "history." Her mental illness. My mother has been prone to debilitating depressions all her life, and this justified our lying to her. For her own good, of course. The way you treat a child.

She scribbled on a dinner napkin a list of questions for the doctor.

"What's going to happen to me?"

He patted her slightly swelling ankles, "You're going to go home to rest."

But at 62 years, she is not such a child as all that. I don't know exactly when she knew, perhaps there was no one moment. But she knows. I'm glad that she has outsmarted the doctor, and us.

▲ ▲ ▲

My aunt, my mother's sister, will stay at my parents' house Tuesday to Thursday to help ease my father's burden. That is the plan now. We have had different plans since finding out she was terminal the first week of August. After all, we have six months left. We will make these months a testimony to life, she will enjoy her last days, we will make her enjoy her last days so that there will be no regrets,

she will have none, we will have none. My sister
and I wanted to take her to Cape May to look at
Victorian mansions; my aunt wanted to bring her to
the winter house in Florida. But the plan has
changed. My mother will not get out of bed.

In the hospital, before the setback that left her bed-
ridden, my sister, the second oldest, and I would
play Chinese checkers with my mother. We would
help her walk to the next ward where they had a
few board games in the lounge. (Against her will,
but they told us she needed to get out of bed—to
prevent pneumonia, after the anesthesia.) We all had
to play with one less checker because the game was
missing pieces. When her pain killer began to wear
off, we'd have to go back. We never did finish a
game.

Back in her hospital room, after we persuaded her
to take another pain killer (she didn't want to be a
"drug addict," she would say, but "she wanted to do
the right thing"), the three of us took a nap. My sister would lie next to her, my mother's "good arm"
(the one with lymph nodes intact) around her. I
would curl up the best I could at the bottom and
hold onto her toes, her "bad arm" resting on my
head or on my shoulder. If they could have left us
like that... But the nurses, the interns. Or my oldest
sister would arrive with her young son.

"Come give Grandma a kiss," my mother would
say, holding out her arms.

But she was afraid, damn her, my oldest sister. A
deep, nameless fear, the one people have of snakes
and spiders and forests at night. Irrational, but still
they won't come near, they won't touch—even when
the snake is harmless to them.

"I blow you a kiss, Grandma, like this, see, I blow
you a kiss," my nephew would say, as my sister's
arms kept him from the arms outstretched to him.

And it is this—hearing the last requests, the last refusals—that breaks my heart.

▲ ▲ ▲

The daughter sits at the table with her aunt, her father. The family spends less time sitting with the mother in the bedroom: she sleeps more; she moans, calls for us to come, tells us to leave when we do. She spends a great deal of time trying, unsuccessfully, to have a bowel movement. These raw physical needs—this is where the daughter is not very good. The aunt and father are better—they are older, they have watched people die before—but even they are not so good at bedpans, not for extended periods of time. The daughter begins to think, but not say, how can this go on for six months? (She does not say this in front of the father because he will weep, uncontrollably, in a way she has never before seen him lose control. Privately she says to the middle sister, there must be less time than the doctors say.)

Because we are impotent to help her, we, instinctively I think, try to help ourselves. We fry chicken, make tea, slice up cake and talk. We talk about ways to get my mother to help herself, and we no longer worry about the volume of our voices. We don't say it, but she has moved to the next circle, one ring closer to death. But we still speak of ways to inspire her. If only we could get her to a support group, where she could talk with other cancer patients, maybe she would not feel so alone. Perhaps the counselor from the hospice we have contacted will help. And then the conversation (although never our thoughts) moves away from the illness, and we speak of easier things: dogs and fleas, sunflowers, baseball, and golf games. Soon bubbles of laughter rise to the surface, are airborne—and then my mother's call pricks them one by one. My father goes to her. "How," she asks, "how the hell," she asks in brilliant defiance, "can you all be so happy?"

Shame? No, it is hope I feel when I hear this. Hope.

▲ ▲ ▲

One aunt leaves, the other aunt comes for the weekend. This aunt lives in Virginia and it has been difficult for her to get here, although she has been trying for quite some time. Now that she is here I am glad, for there is an unspeakable urgency.

No matter what she has been told this aunt is not prepared for what she sees: the jaundice, the cracked lips, the smallness of the body sunk beneath covers and pillows, the dull look in the half-closed eyes. (I vaguely understand, vaguely remember what it is like to be shocked by the unbelievability of it all, but I have adopted my own strategy. The deterioration is tolerable to watch because it is not me watching, it is the other one, my doppelgänger who brushes appearances aside and still urges the mother, refuses to let her have her way, because the doctors have told us: there will be more time.) Still it is beautiful to see them together, these two sisters, sitting in bed holding hands, my aunt brushing away tears with her free hand. My mother and her two sisters have always been close, and she has been waiting for this one. Instinctively I know this, although I can't begin to guess at the significance.

My aunt tells a story. It is about a date my mother went on with my father when she was very young. She emphasizes very young, but she does not say how young, which means it must have been scandalous (my father is seven years older than my mother). It was quite a prestigious outing: they were going to Radio City Music Hall to see Sonia Henie, and my two aunts worked on my mother's makeup and outfit for hours. "What a beautiful girl!" the passersby waiting on the subway platform had exclaimed.

My mother smiles, weakly, but she smiles. In the past few weeks, I have begun to hear many family stories, stories of before my time. The mother gathers what she has accumulated to pass on to the daughter: the legacy.

Since the aunt seems to be in control, the daughter leaves the bedroom and sits in the living room with her father and uncle, understanding that they too need tending, that this process of death is all-encompassing.

For with the aunt's arrival, the mother has slipped even farther away. This aunt has been taken in by the mother's will, this aunt does not insist that she try to get up, try to sit in the chair next to the bed, to pick up her water glass herself. Everyone begins to surrender to this will that was never, ever before so indomitable. Her acquiescence is, in its forcefulness, an act of defiance.

▲ ▲ ▲

When the painkillers' effectiveness begins to lessen, not lasting the full four hours, we bring her the pills more frequently. She objects strenuously, even as she swallows them in desperation.

"It hasn't been four hours yet, it's not time," she complains, the sense of duty, of deferring to those who know best, even now remaining strong, revealing itself in this last vestige.

"It doesn't matter, it's all right," we coax. Or we lie: "Yes, it is, it's time."

Over the phone the doctor tells my father to give the pills as frequently as she needs them to be comfortable, stay at this dosage as long as possible, because once it's increased we can't go back.

We can't go back.

Morphine is right around the corner.

The disease is progressing more rapidly than originally expected. The doctors had planned some chemotherapy. But the plan, once again, has changed.

My father hangs up the phone and cries.

I vaguely begin to understand: there is almost no time left at all. And she herself is snatching it away, claiming it as her own, doing everything she can to hasten this disease along. She will not do what is expected of her. For the first time in her life, she will not do the right thing.

▲ ▲ ▲

The day she was scheduled to be released from the hospital, she collapsed on the bathroom floor. A brain seizure, they thought. Three pints of blood lost through the wound in her armpit.

Intensive care. CT scans. Transfusions. Telephone calls at five o'clock in the morning. Worse than we thought, perhaps, a possible brain tumor.

The daughter thought this was the end. The mother lying in the emergency unit, the oxygen tube in the nose, the good arm puffed up three times its size, every vein collapsed, and the nurses still trying to get an IV going.

The pain is too much. No, we finally say it. You must find another way. They find it, the vein in her neck is opened to receive the blood.

My mother's pastor has come. She is a good pastor, a woman who has the gentle strength of unwavering faith, and she alone seems to be able to bring some relief. Together the three of us pray, although I do not share their belief in this Father, this male Physician, and I feel a twinge of betrayal at the words. But the words seem beside the point, the wafers, the grape juice, I will do all of it, mostly because my mother has not asked me, has in fact expressed concern to the pastor that this is not my way. If she can honor my convictions, I will honor hers. It is a mutuality between the three of us, holding hands, praying, invoking strength that each of us alone does not possess. Perhaps I am rationalizing, but the words seem beside the point.

My mother, although a teetotaller, has always liked the sweet, syrupy Communion wine. She looks disappointed that the pastor has brought grape juice to the hospital. I shut my eyes; it is painful to see her disappointment, even in so small a thing.

But there was no seizure, no brain tumor. A fainting spell due to the abdominal pain. Relief. She will be sent home soon. Only a false alarm. And only a false relief. The wound in the armpit does not heal.

▲ ▲ ▲

Since my mother does not get out of bed, my brother has brought her a phone to keep in the bedroom. It is a touching gesture, one of the few ways that he, as an adult male, can express his love. For he cannot crawl into bed with her, cannot be with her, cannot love her the way her sisters and daughters do. All of that was taken from him long ago. Yet he does love her, fiercely and tragically. So he has brought her this phone. And within days, she is unable to use it. It is this way with all our plans—no sooner are they conceived than they are obsolete.

▲ ▲ ▲

The daughter is not sure the mother even knows she is here today. This is the first time the daughter sees the beginning of incoherence, a wild, unfocused look in the yellow eyes. The father talks to the mother and discovers the mother is aware of the daughter's presence. She is simply not interested then. But the daughter is not offended by the mother's indifference. Somewhere—deep within, where she is still whole and undivided—the daughter understands and is in agreement. She is pleased the mother can take her for granted.

But always on the surface there is the unacknowledged: the fabric of our lives.

The daughter's body moves into the mother's bedroom. The daughter's hand picks up the mother's hand, the daughter's head bends down to kiss the mother's cheek, the daughter's lips say, "I love you, Mom."

▲ ▲ ▲

The aunt wordlessly greets the daughter in the driveway. The daughter's hello smile fades and slowly she begins to understand, but not until she pushes the aunt aside, rushes into the bedroom and sees the corpse—that I become both my mother's daughter and myself.

I cry, not sob, I wail, together my aunt and I scream out the passing of a life. It is myself—no decoy, no double—integrated through the force of the pain I feel, not only of the moment and the weeks before, but of the weeks to come—the unbearable, inescapable pain that will, as inevitably, change who I am and what I may be. It is as one person, then, that I can, that I will mourn the early death of my mother of which she has been both victim and engineer.

For it is late August, and she has died, twenty-five days after her cancer was diagnosed, twenty days after she was given six months to live.

Hostile Takeovers

Naomi Glauberman

The earth shook last night.

I was in bed. I'm almost always in bed at earthquake-time.

"The earth must be angry," I said.

Larry was ready to argue. He thought the earth should be more selective. Why take it out on us? We weren't the ones cranking out poisons and burying nuclear wastes. But that's not the way it works.

We didn't have that conversation right then. Right then we jumped out of bed and raced to the kids' rooms. It was over before we got there. A little rattling, but nothing hit the floor. Larry got back into bed and I went outside.

The Sandowskis—all four of them were in their bathrobes and barefeet. Ellen Kaye and her son Gabriel were wrapped in blankets. Neil and Betsey had run out with their earthquake supply kit and foam mats for their son Matthew who had the flu. An English couple was walking to their car from one of the new restaurants. Altogether there were exactly twelve people at our crowded end of the street and four at the other. It felt like a big crowd. Maybe there were others I couldn't see. People released by that sudden trembling. Squeezed up through the concrete and asphalt for one more look around. Just because I didn't see them, doesn't mean they weren't there. There's plenty of things I don't see. Earthquake or not.

In those days, I thought I could see almost everything. Well, not see exactly, maybe sense is the better word. I do sense things. But I am not very good at

159

sensing earthquakes. They sneak up on me left and
right. And more often than not I am stark naked at
the key moment.

But I know enough to get dressed as soon as possible. By the time I hit the street last night, I was not
in blankets or a bathrobe. I was fully dressed. Shirt,
pants, boots. O.k. no socks under the boots, but no
one could tell. I looked like, and was in fact, the perfect person for neighborhood patrol.

One of the things I did not see, in the days when I
thought I could see most everything, was the tumor
growing inside me. Oh, I knew something was
there. But it did not—even for one second—occur to
me that it was a tumor.

"It's capillaries—weak capillaries," the acupuncturist said, as he stuck tiny needles into my hands and
feet. The acupuncturist wasn't my first choice. I
didn't go to him right away. First I went to the emergency room. I had to. I was doubled over the
steering wheel and cried all the way to the hospital.

"Nervous stomach," the doctor said. "I have this
kind of pain all the time," she might have said. "So
do most people. We live with it."

So much for Western medicine.

Then, I went to the acupuncturist. "Don't worry,"
he said. "You are a person with an amazing synchronicity between your mind and your body. You
have immense powers to heal yourself. And you certainly will." He stuck in his needles for months. I
stared at the ceiling counting shadows while electric
currents bounced wildly through me and congratu-
lated myself on finally becoming a Californian. I was
so busy basking in that flattery about my own special body-mind linkages, I was convinced I would
heal myself right up. I truly believed it. Then the
pains got worse. No one could figure it out.

I thought I could see things. Secret meanings. Deep causes. My mother was dying. She had pains. Blockages. Nothing moved right through her ancient self. Three thousand miles away, my own poor body was mirroring her signals. If I couldn't be with her, I would at least bear her pain. Who the hell did I think I was?

At the time it seemed reasonable enough.

It wasn't.

I might never have known if it weren't for the earthquake. Not this earthquake, the last one.

That was the only earthquake that didn't catch me in bed. Due to my pains, aches, and general bodily failures, I barely slept in those days. Pain held me through the night. I'd finish reading the newspaper hours before the sun rose.

Then it happened. The earth shook. Shook, rattled, and rolled.

I was already dressed, but I could scarcely go on patrol. I could barely move. I was truly sick and no synchronicity between either my own mind and body—or my poor body and the roaring earth—was going to make me well.

It was Max's second birthday. Larry had left for work. Dava carried Max downstairs and we sat on the stoop. Neil and Betsey were drinking coffee and listening to the radio. The skyscrapers downtown had been evacuated, but everything seemed o.k.

"Boy, that must have really shaken you Caroline," Martha Sandowski said, her bathrobe half on and her twins trailing behind her. "You look awful."

I didn't want my misery to be so apparent. I was used to feeling terrible, but I didn't want it to show. I went back to the doctors. This time they found something. There is a polyp, said the young doctor. That did not bother me. I remembered presidential polyps. They came and went as easily as a breeze.

The doctor did not think I had the appropriate attitude. He spoke of my particular polyp in very serious tones. I would need surgery. If the surgery didn't work—who knew what-all was growing inside my body.

My brain was at standstill. Mostly I worried about earthquakes. "What'll happen," I asked the surgeon, before I signed the release forms, "if there's an earthquake while I'm lying on your table with all my insides exposed?"

"Don't worry, don't worry," she said seven thousand times. "If there is an earthquake, we will just stop." This did not exactly ease my mind about power failures, gas leaks, caved in walls and unexpected explosions—and what exactly did she mean by stop? But my bargaining position was not a strong one and I let them go right ahead.

Looks good, the surgeon told Larry after the operation while I slept in peace. Everything looks healthy. She'll be fine.

I was hooked up to a morphine machine and doing swell.

A few days later, the surgeon came back.

"I just got your path," she said.

How nice, I thought, even in the medical profession, that most strait-laced and conservative of groups, they are seeking new modes of expression. They are looking for new and better ways to articulate complexities. To help us put our minds and bodies together. She is about to help me embark on my new path, my journey to ultimate health and salvation. At last my mind and body will be in perfect tune.

"I am shocked," she continued.

Wait. Wait. Wait. A path is nothing to be shocked about. Oh—it might be too wide for some tastes—

too narrow for others—but this could be worked out—we can always go forward.

Something was wrong. We were not east or west or north or south talking the same language.

I was not getting it. She tried again. "Your pathology report. I just got your pathology report from the lab and I am shocked."

That didn't sound good. They had taken away the morphine. My stomach was plastered up from one end to the other. I felt numb, but I couldn't tell if it was body or mind. What was she telling me? What could I hear? She drew pictures on little note pads that were distributed by a pharmaceutical company. She spouted statistics of recurrence and recovery rates.

She was shaking.

I didn't get it. She kept going. She said that an older colleague told her not to worry about the statistics. He was sure I would lead a long life. Still she had to tell me that things didn't look good. Odds were this tumor had gone too far. Poisons may have leaked out. Wild cells might be multiplying deep within. Who knew what corner of my body, what vital organ would be struck next. Oh they could do tests. They could keep checking. And maybe there should be other treatments. Chemotherapy. Radiation. Medical science could accomplish all kinds of miracles. We would just have to wait and see.

This was not expected. But why not? Cancer was an epidemic. AIDS was an epidemic. Starvation and wars were sweeping the world. It was a time for dying before your time. So what if I thought I'd live forever—who doesn't?

The next morning she came back. Half-apologized for being so upset. Said she got herself confused with me. That's what worried her so. I tried to help her out—told her to remember that I was the one

attached to all the machines. She was the one with
the stethoscope in her pocket. She should be able to
keep that straight.

"Oh it's not me I'm worried about," I said. "It's
the kids." The kids are too young. They need me. I
can't go quite yet. Max was just two. He didn't
know what was happening. Fear and the panic of
sudden and irrevocable loss were written all over
Dava's face each time she came to the hospital. I had
thought my concerns might be bigger. Who would
patrol the neighborhood in case of earthquake? Who
would devote themselves to the end of starvation,
wars, and injustice?

The sad truth is, the poor aching troubled world
did not appear in my fears for even one second. No,
it was the kids, just the kids. Max would grow up to
be one of those troubled young men, eyes slightly
downcast, who admits that his mother died when he
was very young, and he can't even remember what
she looked like. I worried about the circumstances
under which he would mumble those lines. And
Dava, on the edge of growing up, the years when a
mother was crucial. I couldn't bear it.

"Don't worry," the surgeon said, "your children
will not be alone. Larry is a wonderful father."

Wrong line. Wrong words. Doctor, dear doctor,
what you are supposed to say is. "Don't be ridicu-
lous, Of course your children will have a mother.
And that mother will be you. Your lifeline stretches
uninterrupted across your palm. You have nothing
to worry about."

"Oh, I couldn't have said that," she said. "It
wasn't true."

Truth. Was it true that if there was an earthquake
while I was on the operating table they would have
stopped still, and calmly waited for the earth to stop

shaking? I have my doubts. All of a sudden, truth becomes some sort of high priority?

She didn't mention my lifeline. Just told me how the kids would be happy with their daddy.

"But a mother. A mother," I stammered, "Don't you think there's something special about a mother?"

The surgeon tried to take me seriously. Her eyes narrowed. She was searching somewhere for the answer that would make everything all right.

"Oh, I don't know," she said, slowly, deliberately, reaching for the truth, "I have some friends whose mothers died when they were very young and they've managed."

It was in December that she told me this. I was out of the hospital but still in a bad mood. They'd recently pulled a tumor out of my depths, and I'd been put in a control group for a study on how cancer patients responded to extra care and attention. I would not be getting any of these extras. At the end of my interview, I asked the counselor—what about the special services. She blushed. The computer put you in the control group—you weren't even supposed to know about anything else. But it was right in the brochure, I pointed out. You must be the only person who read that, she said. I took this as an omen. There was a fifty-percent chance I would survive cancer. There was a fifty-percent chance I would get in the control group. The implications were clear. And now the doctor was telling me not to worry, my children would do fine without me. Was this the way I would go into that dark night? It wasn't quite night, but it was already dark and cold. End of December. Shortest days of the year. The car was deep in the parking structure. I left the hospital with armies of clerks and nurses heading home after office Christmas parties.

That parking structure always makes me think of earthquakes. It would not be a good place to find oneself, but what matter? At that moment, the collective trauma of an earthquake held a certain appeal. No lonely melting away of the flesh.

Weeks later, I returned to the surgeon. The scar, glowing red across my abdomen was angry, she said, but otherwise things looked o.k. I assumed it was me that was angry, not the scar, but that wasn't what I wanted to discuss. "Would you really say that I have Cancer?" I asked. "My interpretation of my case is that I had a polyp which had a bit of cancer, which spread a bit further yet, but that is all gone, so Cancer is not exactly what my particular disease should be called."

The surgeon was tired. She had a cold, and her eyelids were slightly puffy. "I know what you're saying," she sighed, "But what you are describing is, in fact, what we tend to call Cancer."

"And the statistics?"

"Statistics are numbers. They might or might not mean anything. You are an individual person. Take it from there."

Take it where? I didn't know where to begin. I was tired from my surgery. I wanted to stay in bed. I wasn't in terrible pain, all my basic parts were working, but there in the hospital I saw how easy it was to die—nothing sudden, gradually you are just too tired, or too cranky, or too bored—the world would roll on without you, and that would be that.

"I don't get it. How do you live if you think you might die any moment?" I asked the surgeon.

"Anyone can die any moment," she said. I knew that. I was always telling myself that I could be hit by a truck, or fall in the bathtub—so why worry unduly about monthly checkups.

"Anyhow," she went on, "the people who deal with it the best are the religious ones. They just accept it as God's will and go on their way baking cakes and doing their shopping until they're gone."

She didn't advise me to take that route, although I can't say I completely ruled it out.

I was looking everywhere for help. Doctors. Lawyers. Therapists. Betsey, my neighbor told me about a group for cancer patients, called Healthful Happenings. Time was, I never would have given an organization with a name like that a single thought, but times change. When I did call, I explained that I didn't exactly see myself as having cancer, but wondered if their services would be available to someone in my circumstances. They told me to come right over.

Eventually I found my way to a too modern and too high building in Culver City. Everyone at the meeting talked about how frightened they were when they first learned they had cancer, and how much they'd changed since they discovered Healthful Happenings. I had my doubts but was not ready to write it off. Before I knew it I was hooked. I went to meetings and I went to workshops. I went to therapy sessions and art sessions. I was trying to make sense of something. Everyone was.

I joined the Thursday morning therapy group. Scanning the room, I was relieved (embarrassing, but true) to see that there were other people my age, or even younger filling the chairs that lined the walls. We went around the room. We didn't actually move—everyone just introduced themselves. The regulars said their name and their cancer and how much they liked Healthful Happenings. Lewis, the therapist, said he'd never had Cancer, but he's written six books, has been married for twenty-six years, had three daughters, and just bought a big new house, because he's learned from all his friends with cancer that you have to appreciate life and take risks. At the end, new people had to tell how they got there. I told the long version. Tumors. Tests. Mothers. Brothers. I didn't leave out much.

"You've turned all these awful things into a story." Joanne, who had leukemia, was furious when I finished.

"That wasn't so bad," Marvin, recovering from prostate cancer, said. "What was bad was that you smiled all through it."

"I smiled, so you wouldn't worry," I explained. "I smiled to let you know that now everything is alright, more or less."

"I hear you. I hear the words you're saying," Lewis said, "but somehow, I don't feel you're really feeling them. You have Cancer, and having Cancer is really hard, and I want you to feel what you're feeling."

I no longer felt like smiling. They were right. It wasn't that I liked my story, but I did like to tell that tale. And I did smile. I smiled because, as far as I could tell, the worst was over. All those awful things had happened, but I had gotten through, or would get through, or might get through. I smiled so that they wouldn't worry. I'm not sure if this is a sign of weakness, or what.

I couldn't tell what they were thinking. I worried that my sensing mechanism had been cut right out, some form of concentration camp torture. Doctors don't bother themselves about stuff that can't be smeared onto slides. They don't think much about why some people can see things that others can't. Maybe your soul doesn't have anything to do with your brain or your heart. Maybe it's something that floats around your innards, your lymph nodes, your intestines. They cut out what looks like a piece of raw flesh, but there's all this crucial material that they can't see. They don't have a clue that it's there. "Don't worry, you'll be alright," they say. "We got all of it." "All of what?" I should have shrieked. Some of that could have been very important. It was not ready to be sliced off and sent to a lab in an aluminum bowl.

"Do you really think that?" Lewis asked. "Do you often think of yourself as a concentration camp victim?"

"No...it is not an often situation, " I said. I know I was not in a concentration camp—I know I had surgery. But they shaved my body and I lost twenty-five pounds, and everybody in this rooms' hair is falling out from chemical treatments, and it is very hard, if you happen to live in this century, which most of us do, to not occasionally get a little concentration camp imagery caught in your head.

Three women in our group died and two others weren't doing very well. Lewis said this was unusual and unfortunate, but after all, dying was part of living with cancer, so we should accept it. "I heard they were going to disband our group," Joanne said as we poured ourselves herbal tea before a meeting. "People said it was jinxed with so many deaths, but I guess they didn't have another therapist, or another room, so they've kept what remained of us."

It didn't bother me that so many people kept dying. I don't mean that I actually liked that they died. It was horrible how they died so frequently and painfully, but I had to admit, that with my mother having been dying for what felt like a hundred years before she finally died and the surgeon telling me it was important to face my own mortality, that there was something—I don't know—not exactly interesting—but there was something I liked about knowing so many people at the very moment when they were taking leave. I had expected huge cataclysms of emotion. But, in fact, it was . . . ordinary. Life doesn't suddenly get blown up and significant just because it's coming to an end. You put your affairs in order, answer all the letters you'd been meaning to write, and consider whether it was appropriate to settle old scores.

It wasn't quite that casual. We would get furious at the obtuseness of someone's doctor or lover. We would wail at the thought of a four-year-old child losing her mother. We passed the tissue box around nonstop, but still, there was something ordinary about death. We learned it was right there. Always.

My health kept improving and with all of this dying in our group, I found myself listening most of the time. I gave occasional medical bulletins and rarely mentioned my mother.

Then, one day I did.

"I can't believe you've been keeping all this in," Lewis said. "These are stressors. I would invite you to examine how stressful these issues are in your life."

"It's not like I'm not dealing with it," I said. "It's just that here, in this group, there always seemed to be more pressing problems—Joanne's low blood counts, or Corinna's surgery."

"Did you resent that?"

"No, of course I didn't resent it. I just felt I could wait."

"Do you mean to say that you didn't think your story was important?"

"Listen Lewis, I know I am the most important person in the entire world. And so is Corinna. And Joanne and Marvin. The point is that all of us important people cannot talk at the same time. For one thing, we wouldn't be able to hear each other."

"You sound angry to me," Lewis said.

"Of course, I'm angry. Why shouldn't I be?"

"Of course, you can be angry," Lewis said. "But not at us. We're your friends. Why don't you put your mother in the chair and tell her what you're angry about."

The week before, Nadine, a nun who had just had a recurrence of cancer in her back, had put her mother in the chair and started hitting her with a pillow. Marvin was so upset he had to leave the room. He had loved his dead mother and couldn't believe that Nadine could be so angry at hers.

"I don't know if I want to talk to my mother just now," I said.

"If she doesn't want to, she shouldn't. Maybe she's talked enough about her mother already." Marvin said.

Everyone yelled at Marvin for trying to avoid conflict and not facing the fact that he might have some unresolved anger toward his own long-dead mother.

Then we got back to me.

"Sure," I said. "I'll talk to my mother."

"No you won't. It's no use crying over spilled milk," my brother Donald said.

This was a surprise. Donald was not in the group. He was not in the city. Or even the state. He was thousands of miles away, and we weren't on speaking terms.

"Excuse me," Lewis said.

"It's nothing," I said, "Just my brother Donald butting in."

"Oh, I hate that brother of hers," Joanne said.

"We don't want to hear from you, Donald," I said. "So please shut up."

Donald never shut up. Especially when it was required behavior. He kept right on muttering and mumbling and carrying on, while I tried to talk to my mother.

I didn't get angry at her. I never lifted the pillow.

"I think there are things you're not dealing with here," Lewis said.

"I think she's doing fine," Marvin disagreed.

"No Marvin, I'm doing rotten. I can't even get near my mother. The front lawn is too wet and soggy. There are puddles, large puddles of water everywhere."

Lewis hated this kind of stuff, but he always pretended it was terrific. I kept going. I stood up and started walking around the room.

"O.k. Mom," I said, waving the pillow. We were driving over the hill, and everything looked o.k.— the house looked the same.

The green shutters were hanging straight on either side of the first-floor windows. The gray porch stretched along the front, the five chimneys reached straight for the sky. The road was nothing to brag about, and as we lurched along, the group disappeared.

The winter rains had eaten deep crevices on either side of the dirt driveway. The center mound rose too high, and was covered with weeds that bent and crunched under the weight of the car. The ruts in the road were almost concealed by the dense foliage— brambles and briars from raspberry bushes and other thick and wild growing things that clawed at the windows as we drove through.

The grass was high on the front lawn, but the basic contours looked right. We parked the car and headed across the lush grass. Something was wrong. Water gurgled up about our feet. Dark mud squished over our sneaker tops. The swamp was rising. Off to the right of the house it looked like beavers were constructing a dam. The marsh was reclaiming its territory.

We scraped thick globs of black humus from our feet along the stone step before climbing onto the porch, but we still left dark wet tracks on the broad gray planks. The door was locked.

"Those bastards. Do you think they've rigged up some kind of alarm system?" I finally broke the silence.

"What does it matter?"

"I don't know," I snapped. "It would just be embarrassing, if the sirens wailed and the cops appeared."

"Don't worry," Larry said. "we have the papers. We're completely legal. Just give the door a shove."

"You."

Larry pushed and the door opened. There was no alarm. There was barely a latch to give way.

We walked in.

First we heard the voice. "You have just reached The Zimmenfeld residence." The tinny sounds of Farmer in the Dell filled the long hallway. The voice went on "No-one is in right now, but please don't hesitate to leave a message. Speak as long as you want. "

It was Donald's answering machine. Somehow it had gotten stuck—and had been announcing itself for years in the spider-webbed house.

The bats had abandoned the attic and hung in rows along the molding in the long cool hallway. Small nests of squirrels and field mice spilled out of the corners of all the rooms. The fireplace in the upstairs living room appeared to have been taken over by a small family of ferrets.

"Stop," my mother yelled. "Why are you going on like this. You sound like a crazy person."

"It's o.k.," Donald said, "Just another rotten apple in the basket, none of it matters."

Now I was getting angry. "Donald, it's your doing that we're in this swamp and don't think any of us are going to forget it."

"Good, good," Marvin was cheering. "Leave your mother alone. Better you should give it to that rotten Donald."

Marvin was right. Donald was rotten. But still, he was my brother. Abby, Becky and I had kissed his baby feet when they brought him home from the hospital.

"Why are you acting so horribly?" my mother would ask, when we teased our little brother. "Don't you remember how you loved to kiss his tiny feet?"

We didn't remember. And we didn't believe it either. But still, even in those childhood squabbling years, I thought we had managed to eke out some fond feelings.

"I don't think so," Abby would say as we sifted through the evidence. "Donald's been furious at you for years, "at least since Dad died. "

She was probably right. Maybe it wasn't just failure of memory that kept me from the excavation of good times. And Donald certainly wasn't awash in good feelings. We had legal documents to prove it.

Leslie, Donald's lawyer wife was worse.

"I'll tell you," she told Abby, "I used to think my sister Phoebe was awful, but now that I've met Caroline I see how terrible a sister can really be."

"Obvious displacement of hostility," Joanne intervened.

"Of course," Lewis said. "I'm sorry Caroline, but I'm not sure you're sticking to the subject. These are all stressors, and stress *is* the subject, but it is already after one o'clock and I think we better continue with this next week."

I was relieved and so was Marvin. The others were probably hungry, except for Lewis, who ate a cheese, avocado and mixed sprout sandwich during each one of our sessions.

The group stood in a circle, the way we always did, arms around each other's backs, and Marvin, who years ago had been a member of Gambler's Anonymous, led us, as he always did, in the little prayer about God giving us the wisdom to know the difference between what we can and cannot do.

I had wanted to go for a cup of coffee with Joanne, but instead I drove to Santa Monica and walked towards the beach with my mother and Donald, while Joanne headed off with Nadine.

"Mom," I said, "I've really been wanting to talk to you, but we can't have a proper conversation if Donald never leaves us alone."

Something was wrong. It was easy to understand how my mother, despite her death, could be hanging around, but how could I explain Donald's presence. He was a tenacious bastard.

"What's to talk Caroline?" my mother asked. "You know what I meant to do, you know I made a mistake—there's nothing to be done."

"That's what I say," Donald said. "The past is past. Let bygones be bygones. Most important is that we're one family."

"That may be important, but it's also horrible," I said.

"Excuse me, miss, I'm hungry, can you give me something to buy a little lunch." A young man with one arm and stringy brown hair, stepped in front of me as we passed the Post Office. I gave him fifty cents. It didn't bother him that I was walking alone, shouting and waving my arms at one dead person

and another absent one. He probably knew we were
all one family. Or maybe definitions of acceptable
social behavior are changing faster than any of us
know.

Still, acceptable or not, the conversation wasn't
advancing.

"Mom, we'll get back to this later," I said. She disappeared and then, of course, Donald melted away
too.

I continued towards the park. Here, at sunset,
overlooking the Pacific Ocean and the curving coast,
under thick fronds of palms and twisting Eucalyptus
trees the homeless and hungry gather to be fed.
Now, in the heat of mid-afternoon, there were just a
few scattered encampments on the grass, small
groups with bedrolls, backpacks and overloaded
shopping carts. Intent joggers, their lungs filling
with the brown scum on the horizon, were plugged
into their own transmitters as they weaved their
way along the paths. A few old people pretended
not to see the others and two policemen on horse-
back kept their suspicious eyes on everyone.

The ground was firm. On the edges of the park,
near the curb, the dirt was muddy from overwater-
ing, but it was not a swamp we were worrying
about here. A sign, near the fence overlooking the
bluffs, warned that the whole thing could slide into
the sea at any moment.

It was good to be free of my mother and Donald. I
felt glimmers of a future. Maybe I was beginning to
sense things again.

"Miss, you want your palm read?" the woman
asked. Wearing old jeans and a Venice Beach t-shirt,
she didn't look like a fortune teller. Her earrings—
four in each lobe—were crosses and skeletons—not
gold hoops. I was tempted but wasn't brave enough
to have her look at my life line or stare into my

future. I might not have been afraid to ask whether or not I should keep going to Healthful Happenings, but I just shook my head and she walked on.

I wasn't sure if Healthful Happenings was really helping, but I couldn't stay away. At the beginning of each session, Lewis carefully read through the multicolored leaflets, enumerating the degrees and accomplishments of all upcoming events, speakers and special guests and their philosophical positions, He passed out these leaflets and then he read them.

"Lewis, " I said, "this is a waste of time. You must think cancer patients don't have brains. We can all read. We have these leaflets right in our laps and we can read them to ourselves much faster than you can read them out loud—and we'll probably pay better attention too."

"I'm not sure you understand, Caroline," Lewis answered. "This therapy session is only one of the activities we have here. Studies have shown that the most beneficial thing for cancer patients is to be part of a community—and we are a community. It's very important that I read these announcements and that you come to as many activities as you can."

"I know, Lewis," I said. "We all know."

"It's true," Joanne interrupted, "we can all read the leaflets ourselves."

"Could we vote," I asked.

"Caroline, it is not a question of voting. It is a question of community. You know, Healthful Happenings isn't for everyone, and if you object so strongly to our procedures, it may be it is not for you."

I didn't answer. I wanted to cry. I may have had my complaints, and I may have been thinking of leaving, but I certainly didn't want to be told that I didn't measure up as a cancer patient working to control her own destiny. I thought I was a pretty ter-

rific cancer patient. I went to my treatments, I
thought positive thoughts, I did visualizations of
armies of healthy cells mowing down weak disorganized cancer cells—what exactly did Lewis mean?

He finished reading the announcements. He read
that Doctor Vinh, a professor of bio psycho immuno
neurology was going to lecture on his synthesis
between eastern and western medicines. That
sounded good. Of all the activities at Healthful Happenings I had a weakness for the lecture series. The
main thing I liked was that the lectures were scheduled for 6:15 in the evening.

Anytime you leave the house before dinner is
made and served, before kids are bathed and read to
and tucked into bed, you are taking a major step
towards stress reduction. The lecture series was a
legitimate part of my quest for health, but it also
relieved me of some stressful life-responsibilities.

Let them eat pizza. Let them eat frozen blintzes or
fish sticks. I was working on uniting body and
mind. Time and space. I ate broccoli and bean curd.
They would soon have their own chance to balance
life priorities. This particular moment was mine. No
blame. No blame. No blame. You have to take care
of yourself.

"Wait a minute," I sometimes said, as we went
over this in group, "what is all this take care of yourself stuff—aren't we supposed to be part of a
community—and not just this little community that
meets here—but what about the larger community—
aren't we supposed to take some responsibility for
that."

"First things first," said Lewis. "Be married for
twenty-six years and buy a significant piece of real
estate—then you might be able to help the human
community."

Should I argue? Could I?

What matter. Neglecting my responsibility to supply my family with healthful representatives of the four food groups, I left the house at 6:10 for the lecture. I was late. The room was packed. The speaker, Dr. Vinh, was pulling it all together. He would tell us a thing or two. He knew about Western technologies and Eastern philosophies.

Most of the elderly audience, uncomfortable in their straight backed chairs, or standing against the walls, or straining to hear from adjoining rooms, had trouble catching the specifics through the Doctor's thick accent. They didn't care so much about east and west, apart or together. They cared about tricks and were waiting eagerly for the demonstration of breathing and acupressure techniques which might help them bear the pains of arthritis, rheumatisms, and the cancers that were eating away at their bodies.

The doctor had an elaborate chart. There didn't appear to be much west in it. The brightly colored oaktag looked like an eighth grade science project bursting with moods and sections of the body and bits of the universe. It was mysterious. It was complete. I feared it wouldn't hold up in translation. The doctor attempted to explain.

"Each one of these body groups is linked to an aspect of personality," he said. "For example, I am a very sad person. I was born sad because of certain experiences in earlier lives. This led me to have very serious lung problems as a baby and young child. The lungs are linked to sadness."

This sounded a bit like blame. Or misplaced responsibility. In certain corners of the crowded room eyes rolled and nervous glances were exchanged.

Still, the Doctor's voice was soothing—and his intricate chart, color coded spheres depicting body-systems was comforting. A whole new way of thinking. An alternative to the hopeless hard facts the doctors in the white lab coats were always dishing out.

The audience didn't mind. All the languages they were learning since they'd gotten cancer were new to them. And these Eastern words weren't as frightening as those hyphenated lists of chemicals that floated around. The audience was waiting for the trick section, the hints about self-massage and auto-suggestion, but they could listen to this talk of past and future unhappinesses. They'd heard worse.

Not Lewis. In our therapy group, he was a mild fellow, who leavened his remarks with an occasional cluck or two. Doctor Vinh's voice was a soft slur of vowels and consonants, healing in their rhythms, even if we didn't know what he was talking about. Lewis leaped to his feet and attacked with a barrage of staccato syllables.

"Well," He sputtered as he strode to the front of the room. "Well I want to say this is a very special night here at Healthful Happenings. Tonight, for the very first time, in the five years since we have been here, for the very first time, you are hearing the words of someone who has not had his theories scientifically tested. We do not believe in past lives here at Healthful Happenings. We do not believe that you are to blame, in this or any other lifetime for any illness that you might have. You were very fortunate to get to listen to Doctor Vinh, and we thank him for coming, but you do understand this is not what we believe."

I felt stress throbbing deep within. What was Lewis so worried about? Maybe it was Dr. Vinh's certainty that got him. Lewis liked to modulate his theories. "We are not guaranteeing cures here," he would always say. "We are just talking about improving the quality of your lives."

What about poor Dr. Vinh. What about the poor old sick people. The quality of everyone's life looked like it was taking a serious plunge at that very moment.

"Oh, I was furious," I told Larry as I ate the leftover slice of cold pizza. "It may have been relaxing not to cook dinner, but that Lewis pushed me right over the stress and anxiety line."

Larry had no patience for any of this. He would have lasted in Lewis's group about two and a half seconds.

Still, despite my complaints, it hadn't been that bad. Dr. Vinh didn't even listen to Lewis. He smiled quietly deep within himself. As soon as Lewis stopped talking, hands began to wave about in the stuffy room. I thought they were eager to join the debate.

"Excuse me, but I'd like to ask Dr. Vinh, can he give us some exercises that would illustrate these theories," asked a woman in a navy pants suit in the front row. It was clear she had no interest in what medical science had verified or not.

"Oh, I don't know if we have time for any demonstrations," Lewis interrupted.

But the crowd clamored, and Dr. Vinh was persuaded to take center stage.

He explained that since he was particularly interested in the lungs, he would show us a series of movements that would help with problems in that area. We all stood up as he led us through arm lifts and deep breaths and a knee bend or two. Then we sat down.

"Very good," the doctor said. "If you do this thirty-six times each day, you will soon see improvement."

Lewis jumped up. "Excuse me. Excuse me. But I must clarify something—are you suggesting that if they do not do this exactly thirty-six times each day—or if they do do it exactly thirty-six times and they do not feel better—are you suggesting then that something is wrong with them and that they are to blame?"

The doctor smiled. No, he said. No, they do not have to do it thirty-six times. They can do it seven times, and then rest, and if they feel like it they can do some more. If they want to stop sooner, that will be all right too. There will be no blame. No blame at all.

Everyone gave a sigh of relief. The room vibrated with blamelessness and Lewis thanked Dr. Vinh. Before we left, we pushed the chairs back against the wall so the room would be ready for the morning yoga class.

White Flowers and a Grizzly Bear: Finding New Metaphors

Dian Marino

I first discovered that I actually had cancer when I woke up in a recovery room in November 1978. My doctor was waiting for me to tell me the results of the biopsy. Yes, I did have breast cancer. I was 37. Cancer seemed like something that couldn't happen to me, and yet it had. I had a month of radiation treatments and began a long series of checkups with doctors, more biopsies and surgeries. My last surgery was in 1983—a lumpectomy, at which time I was put on a hormone blocker. Last summer, I was nearing the famous five-year marker which would put me into a much better (statistically speaking) bracket. I had a checkup and bone scan which indicated bone cancer in two places. I was put on another hormone blocker and given radiation and the summer to put my life into a new framework "the best we can do is slow it down."

My feelings ricocheted all over the place like some cliched Harlequin novel, except they don't seem cliched when you're in the midst of them. I was afraid, angry, grateful, sad, and a whole bunch of other emotions I couldn't put language to. I remember thinking that I had been a caring person and how could something like this happen to me. My history of involvement in social justice issues influenced some of my ways of talking/thinking about this illness: "It wasn't fair. It's so arbitrary." I cried, wailed, curled up into a ball. I also continued to work. I didn't slow down. Later I could interpret this as a way to deny what had happened, but at the time it seemed like my sanity depended on returning to "normal" as quickly as possible.

Writing about how cancer has affected me is very difficult not just because it brings up complex and contradictory emotional memories, but also because this history is intricately embedded in the relationships I have had with family and friends. In writing, my stories seem simple and clear, but they were not so clear or simple in the moment or even now. Ideally this article would be written by those who have lived with me through this period in my life. My husband and daughters have their own versions of what happens when someone you love gets cancer. My friends also have long histories with my fears, anger, frustration, and even small moments of beauty coming from making sense of cancer.

There is another difficulty that I have only now identified. For a long time I resisted writing about my experiences. I did this partially out of fear of re-experiencing some of the emotional roller-coaster feelings, but also because I am concerned that what has helped me to understand and live more calmly and creatively with cancer may be used prescriptively on other people with cancer. I think that the sense of a loss of control is so great with this illness, that it is time for a great sensitivity around issues of power and control.

In part this writing is a history of some of my major intersections with the medical profession; at another level it is about relationships with myself, family and friends, and with those who have turned out to be toxic for me. There are some clues to the deepening of old relationships and the development of new ones. At yet another level these reflections are like ironic arrows. I am the kind of person who might easily have left these conversations to five minutes before I died; I too frequently gallop with

wild abandon into new landscapes and projects without sufficient time for contemplation and savoring.
From very early on in my sense-making of cancer, I
have tried to speak out as often and in as ordinary a
way as possible about so serious an illness.

It seems to me that the knowledge produced from
this kind of engagement could easily remain in the
hands of the professional class. So I have stumbled
around with words over the years and tried to speak
about problems, responses, speculation, small rear-
rangements, and as humbly as possible. One of
these conversations followed a course I was teaching
about Creative Thinking. A woman came up and
said that she had found a massage therapist who
did something called lymphatic drainage. I had terrible swelling of the arm that had the lymph nodes
removed, so I checked out this alternative resource.
It turned out to be extremely helpful; I continue
with this kind of alternative help. While waiting in
clinics and corridors for checkups, I have visited
with people and found that some are not so enthusi-
astic as I am for knowledge about their illness, for
playing an active role in their health-making.

Death is such a responsibility that I hesitate to
project my keenness to be clearer to understand better onto others who share my illness. I write now
not to prescribe but to describe and wonder aloud
about some difficult times.

As a visual artist and teacher, I am engaged in
many kinds of language. For me, meaning is socially
constructed: concepts emerge out of social landscapes and have particular meaning at different
historical times. For example, twenty years ago,
drunk driving conjured up images of chance and
luck. If you made it home without killing yourself or
someone else that was great, but there were not very
serious legal penalties if you killed or injured some-

one or were caught drunk driving. Now, different
images exist—images that have more to do with
responsibility and intentionality—and the legal consequences reflect and also direct this shift in
meaning. Working from that notion of social construction, I observe that there are some
disempowering frames used within much of the cancer literature. One such example is the use of
militaristic or war-like metaphors. Terms like "fight"
and "beat" and "win the war" are commonplace.
Persuading us to understand our illness in this way
may seem unimportant, but I think that it is worth
resisting and struggling to invent more liberatory,
more empowering metaphors. The militaristic orientation carries more harm than good with it. For
example, I can get into a "war" with my cancer and
interpret myself as winning only if my cancer
"loses" or is "defeated." This kind of thinking simpli-
fies and reduces experiences into win/lose
categories. Within that framework, a person like
myself who has "terminal" cancer has lost. I found it
most difficult when friends and acquaintances
would say after surgery, "Oh, now you're cured." I
often took the time to say, "No, I experience this disease as a systemic illness. It might be in abeyance or
remission, but if I thought of it as a 'cure' I might
stop my healthier ways." People like to have things
fit into these very neat and tidy (having little to do
with reality) categories.

   We need a language of resistance in our struggles
with chronic illness. It is not easy to construct metaphors that are fierce and effective without
reproducing militarism in ourselves. For me, a
deeply healing response has been to spend time in
nature. We also need to not get stuck in opposition-
only frames of reference but to discover/invent
transformative languages and ways of being. This

article reflects some ways of understanding cancer that have empowered me, yet they seem so frail and inconsequential that I am tempted to bolt and say, "Oh, it's too complicated" or "It's been said better by others" or all the other phrases that I use to silence myself to persuade myself that the wisdom we are producing isn't so important.

Sometimes I have to resist the conventional ways to understand and then gradually invent small new configurations. One example of a type of language that is deceptive and infuriating is some of the New Age material that proposes ways of healing ourselves. Issues of power and control are extremely central to this illness. I have learned to respond cautiously to people who suggest I read the latest self-help book. At first, I would go out and get these books only to find that the analysis had a "blame the victim" orientation. Very simply stated, "You made yourself sick so you can heal yourself." So simplistic but so damaging because it fits so well with many of the disempowering patterns of interpretation that are prevalent in our mass media and distracts us from linking the personal with the socially-constructed and -maintained structural components to understand something like cancer. It plays the individualism theme that keeps us disorganized and with a simplistic sense of power. It reproduces the theme of power-over, a kind of domination and subordination theme, that doesn't end up challenging us to rearrange how we relate to each other or our home the environment.

A friend of mine told me about "diagonal reading," taking what makes sense for you and leaving the rest for the critics. Some self-help books, or parts of them, I have found extremely useful—in particular, the Simonton *Getting Well Again*.* I have used the meditation, relaxation, and imaging technique for about six years and find that it gives me an enhanced sense of well-being as well as heightening my senses.

After the initial surgery, I had radiation treatments which were once a day for the entire month of January. The hospital was old and gray, and many of my cohorts were also gray with fear, chemotherapy, radiation. I often wore magenta and other disguises to keep myself walking. There are women who go around to the many waiting areas and offer coffee and tea and cookies. One day as I was approaching one of these trolleys, the woman sang out loud and clear, "Are you a patient?" I was furious. None of her goddamned business and I started to scream at her, "I am, but what a stupid distinction as those who come to support need your fucking coffee too." I went to the head of these yellow ladies and told her to instruct these people to act in a more caring way. It did get my adrenaline running and it cued me to how resistant I was to being one of the "gray ones."

While I was going through radiation treatment, I tried to understand how I got this disease. So I read and asked around. It seemed to me there were many possible explanations for my cancer, heredity (my grandmother had died very young from breast cancer), occupational hazards (for the previous twenty years I had made silk-screen prints using highly toxic paints and clean-up solutions), diet, exercise, capacity to stress myself, being among the first users of birth control pills, plus a host of other potential

---

* O. Carl Simonton, M.D., Stephanie Matthews-Simonton, and James Creighton, *Getting Well Again*, Los Angeles: J.P. Tarcher, 1978.

environmental and social factors. Often I read about these "causes" in separate articles and books suggesting that one or the other factor was the primary cause. I found this a bit immobilizing, so I gradually developed a map that I called "an ecology of possible causes" and began to do something with the dimensions over which I had some control. This was important to how I began to understand and respond with my illness, and often different from how both people in the medical profession and my everyday friends thought about it. My conceptualizing broke out of the hierarchal ladder-type metaphor to a more web-like one and helped me to speak out, because I didn't feel I needed to have a specific map but could elaborate and articulate my own—an open map so that as my experience grew I could alter the map itself.

Luckily for me, I had a doctor who suited my needs as a patient. Before that I had had to change family doctors several times because the doctor would ask me a question, I would answer, and the doctor would disregard my answer. For example, I was having difficulty with my eyes—I saw a wavy line when I got into the car to drive. I went to see my doctor and he asked me if I was under stress. I thought about it and replied "no more than usual with two little ones under three." He then said, "Okay, I'll give you two weeks of Valium." To which I responded, "First, give me the name of an eye doctor, and then I'll check out psychological stress with a psychologist." I went to an eye doctor who found the problem with my eyes in two minutes—my new sunglasses were centered improperly; I also changed doctors. By the time cancer was diagnosed, I had an excellent relationship with my doctor. He trusted me as an expert on my aches and pains and feelings, and I trusted him paradoxically because he was able to tell me what he didn't know as well as what he did know, and would refer me when he was uncertain. He also knew how to cry. When the diagnosis was cancer, he was able to help me see information from different perspectives. For example, he reminded me that surgeons know surgery as a response to unhealth and so advice from the surgeon was reviewed from this critical vantage point. My doctor was able to lay out information from research, from other specialists in practice, from his experience as a general practitioner; he would tell me what was not known, and where necessary he would use his access to the medical profession to consult about my case. He was open to my exploring alternative health support and would solicit follow-up reports from me on those responses to the cancer. For me, it was important to acknowledge the limits of knowledge and to add the dimension of the intuitive to the decision making process. He listened carefully to me and I to him. As the cancer became more complicated and I saw more and more different doctors (perhaps 35 by year five), it became clear that I needed to have one doctor who helped me to manage my history and my future; I had ordinary illnesses in addition to the cancer, so it was good that my family doctor could play this role. It was also important for me to get my doctor's best guess (combination of known and intuition) and know that his opinion was more information for me to use in making decisions.

As an educator, I know that the production of knowledge is a political act and that different frameworks organize interpretation differently. My criteria for a good doctor evolved over time, partially by running into doctors who didn't work for me. As I got clearer about what I needed, not surprisingly I could even get some information from those I didn't totally trust. My criteria emerged out of living through some very difficult times and SLOWLY with others producing, finding some kind of integrated response. I did not begin this journey so clear about the importance of this more consultancy model of doctoring, its development through sense-making sessions has helped me find a stronger way to relate to the medical profession.

One incident that stands out in my mind as a turning point was when I shifted from Princess Margaret Hospital to the Sunnybrook Cancer Clinic. A woman doctor introduced herself as the head of my team (of seven doctors of different specialties). She then gave me a physical exam (number 347) and instead of admiring the many incisions and scars that I had on my body and inquiring who had given me this beauty or that wonderful piece of work, she said "I can see you have been through a lot." She was the first doctor to use those scars as symbols of painful experiences. She affirmed that I had a history and did not distract or try to block those narratives by admiring the "technical excellence" reflected in the scars. I told her that I appreciated her open and non-distractive way of communicating and asked if could she teach her peers to come to people this way. Over the past five years, we have developed a complex understanding of me and my illness. An example of this happened last summer when I wanted the results of the bone scan on the phone because I felt that it had indicated cancer and although I had an appointment in a week, my oldest child was going off to university in ten days and I needed to spend as much time as possible with her. Most doctors would not trace the scan through the system to get the information; even fewer would trust that I was the best judge of when I needed to know something. She told me over the phone information that was not easy to tell nor receive, but this gave me a much-needed extra week to spend with my daughter talking about how serious it was this time.

In the first five years of my cancer history, I had four surgeries for cancer, and my odds for survival were not that terrific. When I asked different experts about what could be known regarding odds they would at first answer ambiguously; as I persisted (in the same session), they would get increasingly precise and specific. Finally, I asked one of them if this was a way to deal with figuring out which patients really wanted to know the specifics and he replied yes. It is called staging. If you ask the same question three times in the same interview, asking for more and more information, most doctors will give you what they know, although some still withhold information. (Lose these characters fast. It is my hypothesis that they are not good learners.) I needed to know as much as could be known. Eventually it enabled me to act strongly to enhance the quality of my life. It doesn't mean that I wasn't overwhelmed and anguished to hear that, for example, the cancer had returned. But having detailed information was one aspect of how I understood myself that eventually helped liberate me from some of the immobilizing and self-destructive aspects of my deep fears, angers, and sadness. At one level, these feelings are always close by, yet mostly I have learned to re-frame them as reminders of my current agenda—to live the rest of my time as creatively and peaceful as possible, to unselfconsciously figure my way through the last part of my life.

Family (hereafter referred to along with friends) and friends make all the difference. How I understand my friends in relation to this disease has also changed over time. Initially, I was surprised, delighted, shocked, healed, by the depth and diversity of responses of my friends. My husband ditched his jeans and dressed in a three-piece suit so as to look like a doctor so that he could bring me a cappuccino and the newspaper at seven a.m. Another friend called me at home and asked "How are you feeling?" I replied "Terribly, I'm depressed." "Good," she said, which caused me to laugh because it was not the expected response, "I thought you were going to avoid this part." Some people never responded, many I am sure out of a fear of saying or doing the wrong thing. For me, people's presence, irreverent stories, and attempts to connect were far more appropriate than no response however well-intentioned. A few people would tell me about a friend who was having this health difficulty (back pains, for example) as part of their way of connecting, and I would find myself wanting to add one small sentence to their stories: "But this disease is life-threatening; I'm afraid I'm going to die soon."

My friends expressed themselves in many different yet all very touching ways beginning with just acknowledging that they had heard. Friends that I do not see except every couple of years called to say just that. It sounds small, but in moments of crisis I find it healing to know that my friends are not denying my most recent diagnosis of cancer or so frightened that they wouldn't call. This acknowledgment warms me greatly.

I also have a fear that the cancer will contribute to a social isolation. That people will—with the best of intentions—feel and treat me as incompetent and therefore gradually exclude me from making contributions. I have a fear that people will feel sorry for me and in so doing patronize and appropriate what energy and intelligence I bring to this current phase of my life. Recently, a person I considered to be a very close friend did just that. He told me that he was in a relationship with me because he felt sorry for me and that I was naive to think otherwise. I felt betrayed and angry that someone I had trusted could treat me in such a cold and clinical fashion. It is one thing to feel sad, but to feel sorry is to distance oneself from the pain in such a way that the other person is objectified and treated as a person of very little agency. People who act that way are toxic, and I will resist being anyone's social work project or charity case.

My friends not surprisingly include me in the most unpressured way in their social and work lives. This unpressured part is important because sometimes I find myself in pain or exhausted or just needing alone and quiet time, and each time I have to call and cancel I am touched by the caring enthusiasm they pass on to me. Many of my work colleagues have responded similarly by both acknowledging and including me in the everyday workings of the faculty. These friendships are important because this theme of the social construction of interpretation is impossible without them. My friends do research and find alternatives, and we discuss them. They share their confusions, their analogous experiences and reflections, and slowly, together we understand a bit more wholly that which we see only partially and sometimes not at all.

Last summer, I had the bone scan and could tell by the way the technician responded that something had showed up on the scan. In the middle of the test (it takes about 45 minutes), he reappeared and said, "You look a lot younger than you are. Do you have any children?" I said, "You went and checked my file." To which he replied, "Yes." So I was pretty sure that they had indeed identified some cancer. That same day I went to the massage therapist who is a person I have come to trust over the past year. I decided that this was a unique moment in my life when I could look into my psyche. I have noticed that when I am very frightened I sometimes have courage to face or to see the unseeable. So as my friend did his work I decided to let go and see what images would surface.

The first image surprised me. There was a field of wild carrots (white flowers composed of many smaller white flowers) surrounded by pine trees. Strolling upright through this field was a humongous grizzly bear. The bear looked strong, confident, and curious as it moved through the field of flowers. At one point the bear stopped and picked up a handful of these flowers, which I knew was essence of Dian even as the whole field was me too. Then I was able to make the bear sneeze and laugh, and I flew back into the ground except for one small white flower head which landed on the bear's shoulder. Together we strolled through the rest of the landscape and into another setting: the desert. The images that flowed from this time all shared this playful, strong, and curious quality. The next day I found out that I did indeed have bone cancer. Almost immediately, my husband and I * began to look for a cottage or a place for me to be still. I sometimes feel my cells vibrating from too much work or not enough sleep, and I imagine that I can see them all jangled and in motion. We looked at many different lakes, and at one point I told Chuck that I had a recurring dream that I needed to spend the last part of my life on a lake surrounded by trees with a beach. This became a guide for us; we found as island that we liked called Cranberry Island, and Chuck had a cottage built. The day after we bought

---

* We have been separated for four years but are very fine friends.

the lot we went to look at it again. Much to my
delight, in the middle of the cranberry bog was a
large patch of white flowers. The lake is called
Kahshe, which I later found out means "healing
waters." So far the grizzly has not come.

Fear of Cancer

Carol Gloor

The seed is buried in our cells,
entangled in our DNA.
In some it withers,
in others flowers.
They're not sure why.

They say
no smoking no fat no bacon no beef no stress
check your breasts your cervix your moles
more fiber more fish more carrots
above all relax

but if you get it
it's your fault.

Cancer can take years.
The salami I eat today will trigger
the tumor they find in 1995.
Each year my face slackens,
my bones stiffen,
and on rainy Sundays
I feel black tongues
pushing through my veins.

I'm very quiet
and my cells whisper,
Listen,
live now.

Afterword

Midge Stocker

In developing the manuscript for this anthology, I sent calls for manuscripts to a variety of feminist publications, because feminist perceptions are what I want to hear, the feminist voice is the one I want to cultivate. I did not seek famous women who have had cancer. In fact, for the most part I did not actively seek particular articles, topics, kinds of authors, or anything else. I have been a fairly hands-off editor. In gathering manuscripts, I decided that before heating up the water I wanted to find out what the temperature is. You may sense that your voice is missing from this volume, that the temperature here is not the warm enough or cool enough for you. You can adjust that.

Cancer as a Women's Issue: Scratching the Surface is volume one of the Women/Cancer/Fear/Power series. Volumes two and beyond will be filled with more women's voices, voices of women who have found alternative treatments, women who are taking political action, women who are caretakers for one another, women who have found new ways of thinking about this disease—your voices. Volume one is only the beginning. Do your part: write about an issue related to women and cancer not addressed in this volume, or elaborate on a point you read about here or somewhere else that you think needs more attention.

To add your voice to the chorus demanding change in the ways we think and act about cancer, send a manuscript of not more than 25 double-spaced typewritten pages to Midge Stocker, Third

Side Press, WCFP Series, 2250 W. Farragut, Chicago,
IL 60625-1802. Enclose a self-addressed, stamped
post card so I can let you know I received your
manuscript, and be sure to include a self-addressed,
stamped envelope with enough postage to return
your manuscript to you if you want it back.

Resources

Alternative Women's Cancer Resource Groups

Mautner Project for Lesbians with Cancer
  P.O. Box 90437
  Washington, DC 20090-0437
  202-332-5536
    Direct services for lesbians with cancer.
Lesbian Community Cancer Project
  2524 N. Lincoln Ave. #199
  Chicago 60614
  312-549-4729
    Support groups; political advocacy; direct
  services for women with cancer and cancer
  histories.
Los Angeles Shanti Foundation
  Emotional Support Services Department
  6855 Santa Monica Blvd. Suite 408
  Los Angeles, CA 90038
  213-962-8197
  Contact: Deborah Openden
    Ongoing emotional support groups for lesbians
  dealing with cancer; additional support groups for
  significant others and the bereaved. Services are
  free.

Women's Community Cancer Project
  c/o The Women's Center
  46 Pleasant Street
  Cambridge, MA 02139
  617-354-9888
    Support and services; information and referral;
  political action; education.

Women's Cancer Resource Center
  P.O. Box 11235
  Oakland, CA 94611
  415-548-WCRC
    Support groups and information resources for
  women with cancer. To make a donation, make
  checks payable to the San Francisco Women's
  Centers, Inc.

Selected Recommended Publications

Bits of Ourselves: Women's Experiences With Cancer.
  Fairbanks, AK: Vanessapress Publishers, 1986.
Brady, Judy, editor. *The Women and Cancer Anthology.*
  San Francisco: Cleis Press, 1991 (forthcoming).
Butler, Sandra, and Rosenblum, Barbara. *Cancer in
  Two Voices.* San Francisco: Spinsters Books, 1991
  (forthcoming).
Kauffman, Danette G. *Surviving Cancer: A Practical
  Guide for Those Fighting TO WIN!* Second edition.
  Washington, DC: Acropolis Books, Ltd., 1989.
Lifshitz, Leatrice H., editor. *Her Soul Beneath the Bone:
  Women's Poetry on Breast Cancer.* Urbana: Univer-
  sity of Illinois Press, 1988.
Lorde, Audre. *The Cancer Journals, 2nd edition.* San
  Francisco: Spinsters/Aunt Lute, 1980.
Lorde, Audre. *A Burst of Light.* Ithaca, NY: Firebrand
  Books, 1988.

Morra, Marion and Potts, Eve. *Choices: Realistic Alternatives in Cancer Treatment.* Revised edition. New York: Avon Books, 1987.

Morra, Marion and Potts, Eve. *Triumph: Getting Back to Normal When You Have Cancer.* New York: Avon Books, 1990.

Mullan, Fitzhugh, M.D.; Hoffman, Barbara, J.D.; and the Editors of Consumer Reports Books. *Charting the Journey: An Almanac of Practical Resources for Cancer Survivors / The National Coalition for Cancer Survivorship.* Mount Vernon, NY: Consumers Union, 1990.

Pitzele, Sefra Kobrin. *We Are Not Alone: Learning to Live with Chronic Illness.* New York: Workman Publishing, 1986.

Sontag, Susan. *AIDS and Its Metaphors.* New York: Farrar, Straus and Giroux, 1988.

Sontag, Susan. *Illness as Metaphor.* New York: Farrar, Straus and Giroux, 1978.

Other books are referred to in articles throughout this book.

Contributors

Contributors to this volume are listed here in alphabetical order by first name.

ADA HARRIGAN lives in Jamaica Plain, Massachusetts, with her partner and two cats. She recently finished her first novel, which includes two fun-loving characters who are cancer survivors. She reports: "I still have an untouched six-month supply of Premarin and Provera. The pills have repulsed me ever since I found out the former was preserved mare's (as in horse) urine. I still get my period once in a while but in between suffer hourly hot flashes which I modify slightly by ingesting a Swiss homeopathic remedy."

BEVERLY LODER is a book editor for the American Bar Association. She is also a freelance writer, editor, and poet whose work has appeared in a variety of textbooks, trade books, magazines, and journals. "Changes: The Before and the After" is excerpted in part from her work-in-progress tentatively entitled *I Ride Faster Horses*, a sourcebook for women with cancer and their families. She currently resides with her daughter Christine in a suburb of Chicago.

CAROL GLOOR has been writing poetry, off and on, for twenty years. Her work has most recently appeared in *Right Brain Review*, *Libido*, and *Naming the Daytime Moon*. She has work upcoming in *Rhino* and *Peregrine*. Her first book of poetry, *Giving Death the Raspberries*, has just appeared as part of the anthology *Troika II*.

HELEN RAMIREZ ODELL was born and raised in Chicago. She earned her BSN at Loyola University. After two years of hospital nursing, she went into school nursing where she became active in the women's movement and became a union representative for school nurses. She served as contact woman for Cassandra Radical Feminist Nurses Network in Illinois for several years. She is currently chair of the Chicago Teacher's Union Women's Rights Committee and works as school nurse at three public high schools in Chicago.

JANE MURTAUGH is currently teaching sixth grade in an Indianapolis inner-city school. Her professional experience also includes several years teaching in special education classrooms and working as an activist with local and state teacher's associations. She is coordinator of the new Health Series at the National Women's Music Festival.

LAURA POST was born a "gifted child" into a "dramatic" New York City family and decided early to become a healer. She reports: "The possibilities visioned led me through an ivy-league education while my father's premature death from lung cancer fuelled my interest in the aesthetic purity of oncology research. Though published in *Federation Proceedings,The Journal of Cell Biology*, and *Biochemistry and Cell Biology*, I became discouraged by the unforgiving competitiveness of the laboratory climate. I turned to medicine, in which I imagined I could carve a path of cooperative and creative health mediation. That the medical culture turned out to be equally—though more patri-/hier- archal was not compellingly apparent to this Taurean workaholic until multiple years of medical and psychiatry training had passed. Now, healing myself and doing wholistic psychotherapy with clients, I have also returned to poetry and to speaking at and producing lesbian-feminist events." Her writing has appeared in *HOT WIRE: Journal of Women's Music and Culture, Women and Therapy, Sinister Wisdom, Coming Up!, New Directions for Women, Baltimore Gaypaper, Equal Time,* and *Philadelphia Gay News.*

MERIDA WEXLER lives between the river and the mountains in New Mexico. She has been creating ceremonies for women for many years. A teacher taught by life, her experience with cancer guides her to new ways of healing. She works for the healing of ourselves and our earth home. And she loves to dance!

NANCY LANOUE is director of Chicago Women's Seido Karate Center and 1000 Waves Spa, a relaxation center for women, which has been providing space for the initial meetings of the Lesbian Community Cancer Project. She is eagerly approaching the four-year anniversary of the end of her cancer treatment.

NAOMI GLAUBERMAN lives in Venice, California, with Russell Jacoby and their two children, Sarah and Sam.

NICOLA MORRIS comes from the Isle of Wight, an island off the south coast of England, and is currently living in Vermont where she writes poems, stories, and essays, and teaches writing and literature at Goddard College.

PORTIA CORNELL was born and raised in New York City. She has lived in Geneva, Switzerland and N. Truro, Cape Cod. She currently resides in a milltown in Connecticut where she watches the river flow. She has taught school children and college students and practiced psychotherapy for ten years. She has had numerous articles published on women's issues; she has also written and produced three performance pieces. She is currently working on a novel about two women trying to get married. She is a practicing yogi, canoeist, and cross country skier. She never rode a horse she couldn't handle, although she's been thrown many times.

RITA ARDITTI was born and grew up in Argentina and has been living in the U.S. since 1965. She has a doctorate in biology from Rome University (Italy) and is a member of the Graduate Faculty of the Union Institute. She has co-edited two books: *Science and Liberation* (South End Press, 1980) and *Test-Tube Women: What Future for Motherhood?* (Pandora Press, 1984, 1989). She is currently an editor of *Issues in Reproductive and Genetic Engineering: Journal of International Feminist Analysis* and is active in the organizing of the Women's Community Cancer Project in Cambridge, Massachusetts.

SANDRA STEINGRABER is a professor of biology at Columbia College in Chicago. She writes and lectures frequently on environmental issues and is the author of "Post-diagnosis," a manuscript of poems currently seeking a publisher.

SELMA MIRIAM turns 56 in 1991 and identifies herself as a feminist, a lesbian, and a Jew. She reports: "I started Bloodroot, a vegetarian restaurant and feminist bookstore in 1977 with other women so that I could integrate my politics with my life and with my means of support. It remains the center of my life." Her other passions include gardening, orchids, knitting, and hand spinning.

WENDY ANN RYDEN is a fiction writer who lives in New Jersey and specializes in teaching developmental writing at the New Jersey Institute of Technology and Montclair State College. Her work has most recently appeared in the short story anthology *The One You Call Sister* (Cleis Press). She reports: "The unexpected death of my mother, Mary, through breast cancer, has been the single most significant thing to affect my writing and adult life. The piece that appears in this book was the first of what has come to be many stories, poems, and other accounts of her death and the way it has changed my life. This essay is dedicated to her memory."

Index

A

A.H. Robbins, 9
Abuse
Abuser
    drug, 83
    sexual, 2, 71
ACT-UP, 91
Acupuncture, 49, 160
AIDS, 6
    activism, 91, 100
    hospice, 137
    prevention, 98
    service community, 102
Allergist, 113
Alternative healing, 47–50,
  52, 129, 136, 160, 185
    doctor response to, 190
Alternatives, 120
Aluminum cookware, 121
American Cancer Society, 9,
  43, 81, 92, 94
    Information Service, 14
    public education efforts
      of, 98
    statistics from, 5, 94
American Fertility Society, 87
Anemia, 39
Anesthesia, 10
    general, 104
    spinal, 116
    trip, 106
Anger, 51, 133
    with doctor, 15
    liberation from, 192
Angier Natalie, 94
Anti-toxics organizations, 101
Antibiotic, 39
    anti-cancer, 37
Arditti, Rita, 85, 103
Asthma attack, 129

B

Baghdad, Iraq, 102
Bailie, Tom, 99
Baldness
    people's reactions to, 64
Bass, Ellen, 71
Bathing suit, 113
Bedpan, 152
BGH, 101
Bhopal, 100
Biopsy, 10, 43
    cervical, 37
    excision, 11, 47
    lymph node, 16
    needle, 11, 104
    as outpatient surgery, 10
    skin, 44
    uterine, 37, 39
Birth control pills, 188
The Black Unicorn, 52
Blaming the victim, 88, 91,
  100, 121, 187
Bleeding, 55
Blood test, 43, 73
Body, control of, 41
Body image, 42, 82
    after mastectomy, 109
Bolton, P.M., 90
Bone
    cancer, 183
    marrow, removal of, 4
    scan, 183, 191
Brady, Judy, 97
Breast cancer, 3, 5, 45, 59, 77
    associated with
      clomiphene, 86
    in grandmother, 144
    invisibility of women
      who have, 63

with lymph node
  involvement, *18*
metastatic, *87, 143*
in mother, *143*
political action
  committee, *21*
in sister, *129*
The Breast Cancer Digest, 13
Breast lump, *10*
Breast-feeding, *148*
Breathing technique, for
  pain and nausea, *44*
Budapest, Z, *51*
Buddhism, *66*
First Noble Truth, *55*

C

Calcification, *10*
Cancer
  activism, *91, 100*
  diagnosis, talking about,
    81
  environmental causes, *88*
  as gift, *54*
  lifestyle risk factors, *99*
  as political crisis, *102*
  prevention, *98*
  specialist, *16*
  victim, *97, 121, 126*
Cancer Counseling
  Associates, *119*
Cancer history, *45, 83, 94, 97,
  191*
  family, *15, 69, 87, 100, 144,
    188*
  influence on later medical
    treatment, *44*
  talking about, *81*
The Cancer Journals, 52
Candle, *50*
Carcinogen, *99*
Carcinogenesis, *86*
Carcinoma of the ducts, *107*

Caregiver, *6*
  self-preservation, *149*
Caretaker, *67, 129–130, 132,
  134*
  helplessness, *152*
Carter, Marian E., *90*
Cassandra, *13, 15*
Castro, Fidel, *119*
Cervical cancer, *37, 54*
  in DES daughters, *42*
Challenge, response to, *63*
Chemical factory, *100*
Chemotherapy, *18, 19, 42,
  44, 62, 70, 80, 82, 115, 129*
  effects on veins, *73*
  fear of, *19*
  rejection of, *37*
Chernobyl, *100*
Chicago, Judy, *49*
Childhood memories of
  mother's cancer, *143*
Children
  breast-feeding, *148*
  of cancer patients, *19, 145*
  choosing not to have, *42,
    148*
  fear about leaving, *112,
    164*
  response of, *108, 117*
  with cancer, *47*
Chinese healing, *136*
Choice
  death as a, *44*
  political, *63*
Cholecystectomy, *41*
Chronic illness, *186*
Chronic pain, *62*
Church, desire for solace of,
  21
Clomiphene treatment, *86*
Co-counselor, *109, 112*
  during treatment, *116*
Coltsfoot, *132*
Community, lesbian, *6*

Control, issues of, *184*
Cookware, aluminum, *121*
Cornell, Portia, *129*
Coughing, *113*
Counseling, *119*
The Courage to Heal, *71*
Cramer, Daniel W., *90*
Crying, *109*, *112*
Cure, *38*

D

D&C, *39*
Dalkon Shield, *9*
Daly, Mary, *51*
Daughter, *19*
Davis, Laura, *71*
Death, *53*
    fear of, *143*
    hastening, *155*
    on one's own terms, *45*
    preparing for, *137*
    process of, *154*
Death toll, *93*
Denial
    multiple personalities as
      manifestation of, *147*
Dentist, *112*
Depression, *72*
DES
    daughters of women who
      took, *42*
    granddaughters of
      women who took, *42*
Deterioration
    of body, *153*
Diagnosis, *12*, *77*
    malignancy, *18*
    response of relatives, *38*,
      78
    terminal, *38*, *149*
    without the word *cancer*,
      89

Diet, *188*
    high-fat link to breast
      cancer, *101*
    implications for cancer, *21*
    Kelly, *115–116*
    macrobiotic, *89*
    products, *102*
Dilation and curettage, *39*
Doctor
    discounting patient
      reports, *40*
    effect of frustration and
      fear in, *126*
    eye, *189*
    managing, *190*
    mistakes of, *48*
    need to change, *189*
    second opinion, *15*, *37*
    visit to, *9*, *15*, *37*, *48*, *69*
    visiting two in a day, *112*
Doctoring, consultancy
    model of, *191*
Doctors vs. nurses, *108*
Dream, *122*, *144*
    after surgery, *109*
Dreaming the Dark, *52*, *58*
Dryness, vaginal, *72*
Dying, *51*
    process of, *66*

E

Eating disorder, *85*
Edema, *38*
Elmhurst Clinic, *77*
Employment, sexist
    paradigm, *6*
Empowerment, *97*
Environmental hazard, *99*,
    188
Envy of people who do not
    have cancer, *110*
ERT, *115–116*

Estrogen replacement therapy, 75
Estrogen-receptor test, 114
Exercise, 121, 188

F

Family
  history, 69
  response of, 192
Family farm organizations, 101
Fat, consumption of, 101, 144
Fear
  of cancer, 144
  of cancer returning, 127
  of chemotherapy, 19
  and courage, 195
  of death, 143
  friends', 45
  of getting cancer, 57
  of hospital, 41
  liberation from, 192
  of mother's death, 151
  of recurrence, 80
  other people's, 39
  in others, 54
  taking pain medication to alleviate, 42
  of the unknown, 137
Feminist bookstore, 13
Feminist cancer movement, 101
Fibrocystic disease, 10, 14
Fighting spirit, 59–60, 62, 64, 66, 68
Fisher, Dr. Bernard, 13, 15
Flu symptoms, 39
Follow-up care, 17
Friend, 39, 50, 69, 119, 184
  fear, 45
  griever's, 51
  needing more than, 75
  response of, 192
Frozen section, 12

G

Gall bladder surgery, 41
Gamma-ray detector, 112
Garbage incinerator, 100
Garment workers, 9
Getting Well Again, 116, 188
Gift, 54
Gland, swollen, 43
Glauberman, Naomi, 159
Goozner, Merrill, 100
Graham, Jory, 97
Grandmother, 15
  breast cancer in, 144
Gray, Elizabeth Dodson, 52
Green Paradise Lost, 52
Grief, 49
Gross, Jane, 94
Group, 126
  alternative women's, 213
  cancer survivors', 43
  civil rights, 101
  dissatisfaction with, 81, 123
  grassroots, 7
  grassroots environmental, 101
  health for women, 122
  incest survivors', 72
  Lesbian Illness-Support, 5
  local American Cancer Society, 43
  support, 116, 118, 152
  therapy, 167
  timekeeper, 72
  Y-Me, 13, 16, 20
Guevara, Che, 119
Guided imagery, 89

H

Hair
  loss of, 19, 44, 62, 64, 82
  pubic, 148

Hanford nuclear weapons plant, *99*
Harper's Index, *94*
Harrigan, Ada, *69*
HCG, *86*
Healing
    desire as tool of, *57*
    emotional, *62*
    New Age, *187*
    psychological, *76*
Healing, alternative
    See Alternative healing
Health insurance, *102*
    See Insurance, health
Healthful Happenings, *167*
Hecate, *50*
Hierarchy, *189*
HMG, *86*
HMO, *11, 16, 18*
Hodgkin's disease, *70*
Homeopathy, *49*
Hope, *60, 153*
Hormone
    blocker, *183*
    replacement therapy, *75*
    treatment during in vitro fertilization, *85*
Hormone-dependent cancer, *18*
Hospice, *137, 152*
Hospital
    fear of entering, *40*
    staff, *41*
Hot flash, *70*
human chorionic gonadotrophin (HGC), *86*
human menopausal gonadotrophin (HMG), *86*
Hysterectomy, *56, 89*
    as cancer treatment, *75*

Hysteria, *40*

I

I Am Your Sister celeconference, *96*
Identity politics, *96*
Imaging technique, *188*
In the Company of Others: Understanding the Human Needs of Cancer Patients, *97*
In vitro fertilization, *85*
Incest, *70, 96*
    memory of, *75*
Income, *7, 45*
Incurable disease, *115*
Individualism, *187*
Insurance, health, *7, 45, 48*
Intensive Care Unit, *135*
Interferon, *43*
Intestinal cancer, *115*
International Commission on Radiological Protection, *99*
Intuition, *150*
Iran, *102*
Iraq, bombing of nuclear power plant, *102*
It's Always Something, *85*
IVF, *85, 88*

J

Jara, Victor, *116*
Jewish ritual, *50*
Job
    starting a new, *81*
    loss due to cancer, *45*
Joy at being alive, *61*
Joyce, David N., *90*

K

Kelly diet, *115–116*
Kelly Foundation, *115*
Klein, Renate, *90*
Kushner, Rose, *11, 120*

L

Laetrile, *48*
Language
    or resistance, *186*
Language transformative,
    186
Lanoue, Nancy, *59*
Le Sueur, Meridel, *9*
Legacy, *143–144, 154*
Lesbian, as single woman, *6*
Lesbian Community Cancer
    Project, Chicago, *93, 102,*
    213
Lesbian Illness-Support
    Group, *5*
Lifestyle
    alternative, *7*
    factor in cancer, *99*
Limbo, *38*
Liver
    cancer, *115*
    metastization to, *150*
    scan, *110*
Lobular cancer in situ, *17*
Loneliness, *119*
Lorde, Audre, *47, 52, 63, 96,*
    98
Loss, *4*
    of breast, *18*
    defenses against, *135*
    of desire to study cancer,
        20
    of hair, *19, 38, 44, 62, 64*
    of weight, *38, 44*
Love Canal, *100*
Lump, *114*
    detection, *103*

Lumpectomy, *15*
    compared with radiation,
        13
    with radiation, *15*
Lung
    cancer, *4, 135*
    involvment in breast
        cancer metastasis, *114*
Lying to cancer patient, *150*
Lymph node, *49*
    examination of, *48*
Lymphoma, non-Hodgkin's,
    43

M

Macrobiotic diet, *89*
Mammogram, *3, 102, 117*
    localizing procedure, *11*
    result report, *10*
    risks vs. benefits, *9*
Massage, *194*
    after mastectomy, *122*
    for lymphatic drainage,
        185
Mastectomy, *3, 12, 15, 47, 60,*
    129, 147
    modified radical, *18, 103*
    preventative, *144*
    radical, *143*
    response of partner to, *18*
    surgeon's urgency about,
        14
Mautner Project for Lesbians
    with Cancer, *93, 101*
Medical intervention,
    unnecessary, *15*
Medical library, *13*
Medical research watchdog,
    100
Medical treatment, *163*
    alternatives to Western, *7*
    destructive effects of, *73*
    experience with, *47*
    indignity of, *38*

Meditation, *21, 44, 55, 119, 188*
    Buddhist, *133*
Memory
    of incest, *70, 75*
    of mother's cancer, *143*
    of time before cancer, *79*
Menopause, *73*
Menstrual periods, *55*
Mental illness, *150*
Metaphor, *186, 189*
Metastization, *4*
    of lung cancer, *135*
    of breast cancer, *114*
Microscopic cancer, *14*
Minamata, *100*
Mind control over body, *44*
Miriam, Selma, *47*
MIT, *110*
Morris, Nicky, *1, 143*
Mortality
    cancer, *94*
Mother
    breast cancer in, *143*
    death of, *48, 147*
    single, *6*
Mullein, *132*
Multiple personalities, *147*
Murtaugh, Jane, *4, 37*

N

National Cancer Institute, *9, 14, 92–93*
    public education efforts of, *98*
National Safe Workplace Institute, *99*
Nature, time in as healing, *186*
Naturopath, *129*
Needle, *11*
New Age healing, *187*
Non-Hodgkin's lymphoma, *43*

Northwestern Memorial Hospital, *93*
Nuclear power plant, *100*
    bombing of Iraqi, *102*
Nuclear weapons plant, *100*
    Hanford, *99*
Nurse, *9, 108*
Nutritional consultant, *116*

O

Obesity, *40*
Obstacle, response to, *63*
Occupational hazard, *188*
Odell, Helen Ramirez, *9*
Oncologist, *16*
Organizing cancer patients, *117*
Orphanage, *143*
Ovarian cancer, *5, 85*
    in DES daughters, *42*
Ovarian cyst, *41*
Ovarian tumor, implications of elevated gonadotrophin level, *86*
Ovary, removal of, *114*
Ovulation induction, *86*

P

Pain, *41, 49*
    alleviation with breathing technique, *44*
    chronic, *62*
    control, *65*
    medication, *42*
Painkiller, *154*
Pancreatic cancer, *64*
Pap smear, *37*
Pappas, Jeannette, *64*
Parents, care provided by, *20, 40*
Passing as cancer-free, *126*
Past, cancer as part of, *79*
Pathologist report, *14, 162*

Period, menstrual, *39, 70*
Permanent section, *12*
Pneumonia, *44*
    after surgery, *151*
Political response to cancer, *91*
Post, Laura, *135*
Power, regaining full, *62*
Power-over, *187*
Prevention
    of AIDS, *98*
    of cancer, *98*
Princess Margaret Hospital, *191*
Priorities, *126*
Prophecy, self-fulfilling, *82*
Prostate cancer, *5*
Prosthesis, *63*
Psychiatrist, *135*
Public education, *98*
Public library, *13*
Public perception of cancer, *94*

Q

Quadrantectomy, *14*
Questions, list of, *115*

R

Racism, *136*
Radiation, *3, 14, 38, 54–55, 110, 188*
    as alternative treatment, *12*
    compared with lumpectomy, *13*
    ionizing, *99*
    with lumpectomy, *15*
    side effects of, *38, 47*
    specifics of treatment, *38, 111*
Radioactive isotope, *112*
Radiologist, *16*

Radner, Gilda, *85*
Range of motion, regaining after surgery, *61*
Reach for Recovery, *61*
Reaction of other people, *39*
Reconstructive surgery, *63*
    See surgery
Recovery, *40*
    from sexual abuse, *71*
    strength required during, *45*
    from surgery, *42*
Recurrence, *45, 79, 82, 89*
Refinery, *100*
Relationship, support of, *12*
Relatives
    not telling, *38*
    telling, *78*
Relaxation, *89, 119, 121, 188*
    tape, *129*
Reminiscences of the Cuban Revolutionary War, *119*
Remission, *44, 116, 127*
Resistance, *186*
    Chilean, *116*
Respiratory disease, *114*
Risk, *99*
Ritual
    creation of, *50*
    Jewish, *50*
Rowland, Robyn, *90*
Rush-Presbyterian-St. Luke's Medical Center, *16*

S

Sadness, *192*
Saturday Night Live, *85*
Scar, *83, 109, 110, 166, 191*
Scare
    cancer, *45*
Schink, Dr. Julian, *94*
The Second Seasonal Political Palate, *49*
Second opinion, *37*

Secret, cancer as a, *144*
Seizure, grand mal, *56*
Self-hate, *75*
Self-preservation of
  caregiver, *149*
Sex, *72*
Shakespeare, *133*
Shame
  about breasts, *144*
  lack of, *149*
Shock, *147*
Sibling, *71*
Sidney Farber Center, *115*
Simonton, *116, 118, 188*
Skin cancer, *44*
Sojourner, *5*
Solstice, *56*
Sorrow, *50*
Speculum, *70*
Spirit
  fighting, *59–68*
  non-quitting, *65*
*Stage V: A Journal Through
  Illness, 5*
Staging, *192*
Starhawk, *52*
Steingraber, Sandra, *91*
Stocker, Midge, *1, 199*
Stomach cancer
  confusion with ovarian
    cancer, *87*
Stomach pain, *160*
Story, horror, *123*
Strength, regaining after
  surgery, *61*
Stress, *82, 188*
  as cause of cancer, *47*
  reduction, *119*
Study, loss of desire to, *20*
Superovulatory treatment, *86*
Sunnybrook Cancer Clinic,
  191

Support group, *80*
Support network, *102*
Support services, *45, 213*
Surgeon, urging
  mastectomy, *14*
Surgery, *40*
  accident during, *60*
  gall bladder, *41*
  HMO approval of
    outpatient, *11*
  outpatient biopsy, *10*
  reconstructive, *3, 63, 83*
  recovery from, *40*
Survival rate, *15*
Survivor
  cancer, *96*
  incest, *96*
Sweatlodge, *54*
Swift, Richard, *100*

T

Taboo, lifting of in group, *80*
Tamoxifen, *18*
Tense problem, *38*
Terminal diagnosis, *186*
  See Word usage
Test
  estrogen assay, *11*
Tests
  medical, *41*
Therapist, *50, 75*
Three Mile Island, *100*
Throat cancer, *2*
Time
  caught in, *105*
  decision making, *13*
Times Beach, *100*
Toxic waste dump, *100*
Toxicity of chemotherapy, *43*
Tracheostomy, *137*

Treatment, medical
    See Medical treatment
Tumor
    abdominal, *148*
    doubling time of, *14*
    liver, *150*
    solid, *14*
    in spine, *124*
Twelve-step meeting, *72*

U

University of Illinois
    Women's Health
        Exchange, *13*
Uterine cancer, *5*

V

Valium, *189*
    intravenous, *11*
Veins, collapse of, *73*
Victim
    blaming the, *88, 91, 100,
        121, 187*
    See word usage
Victimization, *97*
Vietnamese healing, *136*
Violence, *55*
Visualization, *44, 74, 89, 121,
    129*
Vitamin therapy, *132*

W

Wainwright, Sonny, *5*

Wallis, Claudia, *94*
Warriorship, *66*
Weight
    gain, *39*
    keeping on, *21*
    loss, *38, 44*
Weil, Simone, *54*
Welch, William R., *90*
Wellness Community, *89*
Wexler, Merida, *53*
Wholeness, *126*
Wig, *20, 64*
Wilder, Gene, *85*
Winnow, Jackie, *6, 95*
Witch recipe, *49*
Womb, *57*
Women with cancer and
    cancer histories, *97*
Women's Cancer Resource
    Center, Oakland, *93, 95*
Women's Community
    Cancer Project, Boston, *93*
Word usage, *96, 99, 115, 121,
    126, 186*
Writing, difficulty of, *184*

X

X-ray, cumulative effect of, *10*

Y

Y-Me, *13, 16, 20*
Yale Medical, *49*